Surviving Surgery
Photographs From A Life

Bernard Gardner, M.D.

Dedication

To my wife Joan, who has always stood by me and supported my dedication to my patients. To my patients, who trusted my decisions.

This book is part memoir, as I recall the details, and part instruction manual for patients about to undergo an operation.

Table of Contents

PREFACE

The patient planning to undergo an operation or in an emergency room, told that surgery is necessary, is often overwhelmed with fear, usually uneducated in medicine and at wit's end about what might be involved. The surgeon's job is not only to make the correct decisions and perform the operation faultlessly, but to allay these fears and uncertainties. Spending the time to speak with the patient and to explain all aspects of the procedures to come, in my opinion, contributes significantly to a successful outcome. This should be done in the office for elective procedures and at the bedside for both elective and emergency operations. This should be done by the surgeon and not by a nurse or resident or a partner. It doesn't matter how busy the surgeon might be.

I'm going to take you on a tour of surgery as it developed in the 1950's through 2000. My intimate involvement in training, academia, private practice in one of the largest private hospitals, research and interaction with students, residents, colleagues, deans and patients will provide intimate details of developments during this period. Changes throughout these critical years reflect on many aspects of surgical practice today. Appreciation of this history will help to interpret why alteration in surgical training is a "hot topic" among today's surgeons.

Scattered throughout these early chapters are comments which are pertinent to patients today.

I have decided to keep anonymity regarding questionable actions of physicians and surgeons to obviate embarrassment. All opinions are my own. All the activities were part of my experiences and interpretations and I am not adopting a "holier than thou" attitude. We all make mistakes, but sometimes motivation needs to be addressed.

A BRIEF OVERVIEW

Many nights I lost sleep worrying about patients and I always felt that I had made the right decisions. I once slept in an ICU bed next to a patient from whom I had removed a large segment of the liver. In the following days the nurses were convinced she wouldn't make it. I brought her back to the ICU several months later fully recovered to thank the nurses.

I had a call from an old patient who wanted to transfer her mother from a hospital in South America where a diagnosis of acute appendiceal rupture was made.

I told her to come. I got a call from the senior resident at 3 a.m. that the patient was admitted and was in good shape, no need to come in to see her. I came in immediately and found that she indeed had a ruptured appendix and operated that night.

On one occasion I got a call from a medical patient of a gastroenterologist who left town and gave the patient my number because he trusted my judgement.

I feel that many surgeons go through similar experiences so I didn't include them in the book.

My father said to me before I left for college: "Don't ever forget the poor people." I never charged or sued a patient who couldn't afford to pay.

I graduated from medical school in 1956. The internship matching program was introduced about a year earlier. The previous system consisted of students applying to many hospitals for internship appointments. This was followed by interviews and a selection process. It was a disaster. On a certain day in March, the selections were to be made and every senior scrambled to contact his (her) first choices.

Can you imagine a single day when thousands of students were fighting for phones trying to get through to training directors, while some directors were trying to reach selected students? (No Apple cell phones in those days.) It was totally chaotic, with hospitals trying to get their best choices while making deals with others to stand by until all was settled. Many hospitals and students were disappointed in their final choices. Hospitals selected in order to be certain of getting someone, and students to be sure to get in a program.

The new matching plan obviated the confusion by having the hospitals list the candidates in order of choice and the students doing the same with the hospitals. The lists were matched and theoretically the hospitals got the highest choice among the students that listed them and the student got the highest choice of hospital that would accept him (her). Aside from an occasional cheating director, where coercion played a role (list me first and I guarantee you a spot in the program), the system was a vast improvement.

The best programs still were in demand and this resulted in very low pay, sometimes room and board with no money. Some hospitals tried to attract interns by offering salaries of $400 per month in addition to room and board. This was very high pay in those days. We traveled for interviews to hospitals that offered these premium salaries. In order to enhance the appearance of their teaching programs, some hospitals described multiple teaching conferences in elegant brochures. Sometimes, we later discovered, a teaching conference might consist of two surgeons meeting in a hallway. Many interns subsequently discovered the myths of the teaching conferences. Most of the time, even if one were held, the intern was needed elsewhere (usually to hold retractors in the OR), or was too tired to stay awake. The best "teaching" services were at university hospitals, where you learned by working with first-class residents. Those programs were still in demand despite the low pay.

States required a clinical year of training after graduation for eligibility to take a state or national board examination which, when passed, permitted you to practice medicine and surgery. That year could be spent rotating through several medical and surgical services or dedicated to a straight medical or surgical teaching experience. The year was called an internship, or as part of further training PGY (post graduate year) .

During those times after internship, one could be drafted into the military services as a general medical officer. Deferrals for one additional year of training were allowed and then you entered with a D rating, guaranteed to spend all your time in your specialty (ranked as a captain). If you went on to a complete residency you got a deferral (5 or more years in Surgery, less in Medicine) and entered as a Major. All the deferred time was paid back, year for year, on active duty.

I had trained for two years in surgery before going into the Air Force. The first year was spent at a large city hospital in New York. There were eight of us that started a straight surgical internship, four of us continued in surgery after that year and the others dropped out to enter a different (easier) specialty. The internship year was a punishing experience, remarkable for working12 to 20 hours a day and little sleep.

After my military duty I returned to residency, spending a year doing research and then completing my residency in California. Successfully completing a residency made you eligible to take a board examination which, when passed, made you Board qualified. Note the difference in those terms when seeing a specialist. Some hospitals require that specialist practitioners (i.e. surgeons) be board qualified, some do not.

Since passing the national boards after internship enabled you to practice medicine and surgery, it was possible in some rural areas to be operated upon by a doctor who had not spent a day in surgical training.

In 1965 I returned to New York as assistant professor of surgery. I became a fellow of the American Cancer Society and subsequently won a five-year Markle Scholarship, which helped pay for my research until I was awarded a number of grants. Through membership in multiple societies and presentation of scientific and clinical papers at meetings, I managed to rise to leadership roles. Some of these activities will be described in detail. I co-edited three textbooks and multiple studies on cancer. While teaching and research occupied much time, the bulk of my efforts were directed to care of patients with cancer and teaching surgical residents the techniques of multiple operations.

The final chapters of this book are devoted to a description of the steps that should be taken before an operation is performed, and the types of medical personnel a patient is likely to meet during the hospitalization. Chapter 9 is devoted to describing things patients should consider prior to operation.

CHAPTER 1: EARLY TRAINING

When I arrived early on July 1, I was assigned to take care of thirty-five surgical patients. They consisted of patients recently operated upon, some awaiting OR time, a variety of extremity infections, intra-abdominal conditions (pancreatitis, cirrhosis, etc.) as well as peripheral vascular disease (ulcers and impending gangrene) and other surgical problems. There was no stress on early discharge in those days, so many patients occupied beds waiting for discharge or operation or for something to heal. Many of these patients were indigent, and had no other source of medical care.

A PGY 3 resident was assigned whose job it was to oversee my fluid and medication orders on morning rounds. He wasn't often available to help with the intern's work. After all, he had been through this monstrosity himself, and now it was my turn.

The head nurse lectured me, on my first day, telling me that she was the boss and I'd better stay out of her way. She was an Italian girl with years of nursing experience and had seen interns come and go. She was a Bellevue graduate, totally dedicated to her patients, and not likely to let some intern screw things up. She was assisted by LPNs (see later chapters) and students at various levels. It was her responsibility to see that all the doctors' orders were filled and care administered. Actually, I learned a lot from her. She had a great sense of surgical problems and knew when things weren't going right. Years later, I transferred my respect for her to many other nurses with whom I worked, even as professor and director of a service.

As the intern on the service, she expected me to be available for any problems, and as long as I worked hard and came when paged we got along fine. She also worked long hours, arriving before morning rounds at 6:30 a.m. and leaving well after giving report to the 4 PM shift.

Would you like to see a list of chores?

In those days, the interns did many non-medical jobs in a greatly under-financed hospital treatment. We worked up all the admissions with a complete history and physical exam (including a pelvic and rectal examination), wrote all the orders, started all our own IVS, drew all blood for lab tests, did all the dressings, helped in the emergency room for surgical emergencies (new admissions were initially seen by the PGY2or3 on duty), transported the patients to x-ray or the OR. (There were no transporters at many hours.) At night, we even cross-matched blood for the emergencies when the blood bank closed early. We often had patients with intestinal obstruction, while another was bleeding from a gastric ulcer. That meant you spent all night between the x-ray department, OR and blood bank. We were on call every other night and weekend, but we often made evening rounds after dinner, which meant you didn't get off until 8 PM on your night off and had to be back for 6 a.m. rounds the next day.

This was charity care and it worked because interns and residents were well-trained and all patients were "teaching cases." On a surgical service, decisions were approved by advanced residents, and the chief resident was informed. and He had the final say about each treatment choice. Attending doctors (those in private practice) did their supervision by telephone in contact with the chief resident (in his fifth or sixth year of training). They did not usually operate with the chief (direct supervision) unless the patient was scheduled for an elective procedure on a mutually agreed to time. There was no Medicare or Medicaid in those days, just uncompensated care.

Patients requiring emergency surgery were operated upon by a resident, selected by the chief resident, who usually scrubbed on the case, after phone consultation with the attending. This persisted throughout my training. Hospital reimbursement was from the state or city, charity (tax) funds or assessments on private insurance, when available.

On a typical day the residents met for breakfast at 5:30, and after 6 a.m. rounds, those of us that weren't scrubbed did our patient care. This meant changing dressings on eight or nine patients, examining the post-operative patients (lungs, abdomen, extremities), and writing notes (chart rounds). Laboratory bloods were drawn by us three times a week and picked up by messenger service and delivered to the lab some two blocks away. If emergency tests were needed, or, as often happened, the previously drawn specimen was lost or dropped by the messenger, we redrew them and carried them to the lab ourselves. We were responsible for washing the glass syringes and stainless-steel needles and placing them in the sterilizer. The barrels and plungers were numbered so that we could match them up when the sterilization was finished. (I saw the same system in China twenty years later, still using glass syringes and steel needles). Then we checked IVs and restarted new ones. IVs constantly infiltrated at night. This was due to the rigid needles cutting through a vein, and it was the intern's job to restart them that night. Our service taught that if an IV was ordered, it had to be given. Today plastic catheters are threaded into a vein and are usually unaffected by a patient's movements. There are IV teams in most hospitals trained to do this. Occasionally there are "pick" teams who bring a portable sonogram to better identify veins.

I'm not finished.

We also tested the urines from diabetic patients (collected by the nursing staff) for glucose and acetone four times a day and wrote or altered insulin coverage. If we scrubbed on a case, there was cross-coverage for emergencies, but usually we got our routine work done before or after the operation. It all depended on organization and keeping an accurate notebook for everything that was required for the day. When a resident made a suggestion, you wrote it in your notepad to be certain it got done. Large pockets were helpful for carrying adhesive tape, clamps, and various other items that might be handy for dressing changes or removal of various tubes.

This sounds like a grueling schedule. It was. But I need to comment a bit about what it did for me. By working up so many patients, I learned the value of a good history and physical examination. I learned a lot about the presentations and nuances of surgical diseases. Years later, when a diagnosis was not confirmed on a CAT scan or x-ray, I saved a number of patients from disaster by treating them according to my evaluation which I trusted.

One example was a 33-year-old woman with deep jaundice. Her mother called me and pleaded for me to accept her at the University Hospital. She had been treated for weeks for hepatitis at a good local hospital. Her hepatitis titers were positive and her CAT scan (in the early days of this technique) was read as showing a normal gallbladder and common duct. But her history started with fever and abdominal pain, not with a viral prodrome: (flu like ague, loss of appetite, early fever). It was a classical history for gall bladder disease: (abdominal pain, vomiting, tenderness, late development of fever). I operated against other medical opinions and found a gallbladder and common duct filled with hundreds of tiny stones. She recovered. I don't mean to belittle the value of our current diagnostic tests, which are wondrous, but to indicate that they should be evaluated in the context of what is clinically apparent.

Another case was a 19-year-old man with sudden onset of shortness of breath, chest pain and a physical exam revealing decreased breath sounds in an upper lobe but with resonance on percussion, findings indicative of a pneumothorax. I sent him for an emergency x-ray and the radiologist called me to say the film was negative. I told him to take another look. A diagnosis of pneumothorax with collapsed lung was confirmed.

I ate lunch early in those days so I could grab a short nap before clinics. We covered surgical, vascular, post-operative and new patient clinics, which usually ran from 1–3 p.m. The city had a large population of derelicts and homeless who inhabited the avenues and other areas near the hospital. These men (rarely women) developed venous ulcers at their ankles and brawny edema of their legs, and showed up regularly at our foot clinic. We learned a lot about venous insufficiency and treated these folks with various colored antiseptic solutions, painting them green or red on different days. (It didn't change the healing propensity.) On occasion, we would apply Unna boots (a weak plaster that hardened) or ace bandages when available. Actually, the only treatment that worked well was to wash the ulcer with antiseptic soap and have the patient keep the legs elevated during the day. This, of course was impossible, unless the patients were admitted to the hospital, a treatment reserved for the worst cases.

The ulcers usually healed only to recur months later after discharge.

Occasionally the police would bring us some fellow who was found lying in an alley with maggots on his ulcers and lots of lice or with frostbite. We often recognized him from the clinic.

After clinics, we worked up admissions and prepared patients for the next day's OR schedule.

This meant seeing that admission labs were recorded on the chart, (often done by us), and that a sample of blood made it to the blood bank. We rounded up the day's x-rays and lab results in order to facilitate evening rounds. After dinner, at 6 p.m. we gathered for evening rounds where most of the teaching was done by the chief resident and other residents at the patients' bedsides. This was a marvelous experience, with the residents testing our knowledge and recommending current journal articles. We visited every patient on our service. We were off alternate nights and alternate weekends, which time we used for reading and study, when we could stay awake.

Night call was tough. The telephone rang incessantly, and usually meant a trip to a patient's bedside to evaluate a fever or restart an IV. By listening to post-operative patients' chests daily, I soon learned to diagnose serious pulmonary complications and to differentiate them from fevers caused by wound or urinary tract problems. New admissions at night usually meant major surgical emergencies, such as intestinal obstructions or bleeding ulcers, and you could forget about returning to your room that night. But seeing and managing these patients acutely gave me a world of experience which I could never duplicate. Working at the bedside of a critically ill patient provided knowledge I couldn't get from a textbook, especially if you worked beside a knowledgeable senior resident.

We weren't allowed to operate on a patient for the first four months of our internship year, although we assisted on many cases, and learned to tie knots by practicing on bedposts or chair-backs. When one of my colleagues was told he would be doing a hernia repair (under supervision) the next day, all the interns sat up with him for hours reviewing the anatomy and procedure to make sure he knew everything about the proposed operation. These were described in a standard atlas of operations. One mistake and we wouldn't operate for several more months.

He did fine and after that we were regularly scheduled for hernia repairs, hemorrhoidectomies, and appendectomies under strict supervision.

All of this was for $40 per month, a room, free laundry and all you could eat at three meals and a midnight snack. The food was the best and tastiest and at the city hospitals it was served by waitresses. I was married at the time and my wife, Joan, often ate dinner with us at the hospital. We couldn't afford to do it any other way.

Our division was run by a famous New York private surgeon who had dictatorial command over our existence. I'll never forget one fourth year resident who was dismissed on the spot for being late for grand rounds in spite of being up all night with a bleeding patient.

Our chairman didn't accept left-handed residents because he wasn't comfortable with them in the OR. He also believed that everyone would be better off being in a second marriage (he was). This worried Joan. Some of us were fearful of his wrath. One day he yelled at a resident "What's wrong with you? Can't you see straight?" and the poor guy spent his weekend off getting eye examinations.

This type of totalitarianism was not unusual for surgery in those days, or in fact in many programs even today. Often a resident was not treated like a colleague but rather as a slave. Our chief owned multiple old Packards, and his chauffeur would drive him up to university hospital at 6 a.m. every morning (he didn't operate at our hospital) and the residents would line up at the door to greet him. That meant they had to make rounds on all his many patients at 4:30 to be finished in time, and make certain all was well and all the IVs started. The chief needed a full report when he arrived. Much of this behavior still exists in some surgical programs today, either by the director or senior staff.

When I got my appointment at Mount Sinai for my second year, the only comment the chief had was: "I guess he wants to be around his own people (Jews)."

Commentary

Although the internship year was hard and strenuous it passed rapidly, and those of us that continued our surgical training never regretted a minute of it. Even on nights with little sleep, each new patient presented problems and treatment choices which we made, and were corrected by a supervising resident. We reviewed each x-ray and lab test until we became proficient in diagnosis. Those of us that continued in surgical training were totally immersed in the surgical discipline. We rarely complained about the long hours; we did what was expected. The chief resident (in his fifth year of training) had final responsibility for the patient's care and it was the assistant resident's job to keep him notified of every problem. The chief resident made rounds by himself daily, seeing every patient and confirming every decision. This was a habit that stayed with me when I became a chief resident. The program was pyramidal, that meant not all the residents got to be chief at in our hospital. Some were sent to other affiliated hospitals to get their operative experience as chief resident.

We were often physically tired and sleep deprived, but were never in a position to harm a patient because of resident supervision. I can't ever recall a situation where I felt that I made an error due to being overworked. As we will see later, this type of supervision didn't always exist on other surgical and non-surgical services.

In those days, coverage by surgical faculty (called attending physicians) only extended to operative cases or seriously ill patients. The chief resident could choose the attending, under whose jurisdiction he would operate, assuming he or she was in town. In my chief year, in another program, things were quite different, and they are very different today. (See later comments on surgical hours today.)

In another surgical division at our hospital, the attending physicians were full-time, paid university faculty and usually available to cover the resident program. Medical students were assigned and did the daily lab work such as blood counts, but not chemistries. The residents usually had coverage in the OR by the faculty. Private cases were still operated upon in other hospitals, and the level of resident care varied widely depending on which faculty member was assigned.

I worked in a charity hospital. Patients were usually indigent or uninsured and often were admitted in an advanced stage of disease. This is often the same today when patients do not have insurance that provides office care allowing earlier diagnosis and prophylactic testing and treatment. We didn't have ICUs, IV teams starting fluid treatments, lab techs drawing blood for testing or transporters taking patients for special tests, all of which subsequently became available in most hospitals in the United States.

CHAPTER 2: THE SECOND YEAR

The hours at my new hospital weren't much different, except I was making $70 per month now, and I had interns (PGY1) doing the initial workup. Joan, fortunately, was working as a legal secretary and making $100 per week, which enabled us to have our own apartment in the city.

The apartment was on 74th Street near First Avenue in an old five story walk-up. We had a bathtub in our kitchen which also served as a counter when covered. I took my showers at the hospital, and Joan visited her parents in Queens when I was on call. There was a living room that looked out on 74th Street, and frequently we got the smoke and smells coming up the street from a Con Edison plant at the edge of 74th and the East River. We had to buy a fan which we turned to blow out toward the street.

You walked down a long hall which counted as an additional room. We put a pipe down the length of this to act as a closet. At the end of the hall was a tiny bedroom and a tinier toilet. There was a window overlooking a courtyard and we had a variety of neighbors. One Chinese family hung cabbage out on a clothesline strung across the court. The smells were wonderful.

Many countries of the world were represented in that neighborhood. Every month there was a parade in the area and we recognized our Greek or Polish or Oriental neighbors.

We went back years later after we returned to the east, and the landlord had realized the benefits of the real estate boom. The old walk-ups had been torn away and replaced by expensive high-rise apartments and condos—with elevators. Our street had become a fashionable residential neighborhood. Con Edison was still down the street, however.

Even though interns were working under me now, I wasn't going to let them be on their own. I spent many long nights working up patients with them. We still did much of the transport work, IVs and basic patient care, but at least we didn't have to cross match our own blood. The hospital was the home of the founder of blood groups and prided itself on its blood bank. As a matter of fact, there were so many doctors rounding and studying things, you could hardly find a patient who didn't have his own study group. This was high class medicine in a high-class hospital!

Some of the older internists did not want to refer patients until all non-surgical treatment was exhausted. This attitude may have stemmed from the days when surgeons ruled the hospital and made many decisions. They were the drawing cards and had the ear of the trustees. One of these fellows, rumors said, was an absolute tyrant and may have driven an assistant to seek psychiatric care. Although I couldn't believe some of the stories, since they dated back thirty years or more, nevertheless it was clear that there may have been some animosity between the services.

While I was there, we had a few surgeons who drove our academic chief nuts. One of these was the surgeon (we'll call Dr. Gross) with the highest income in the United States. This meant he had to do five operations every day of the year except weekends. This he did, and still had time left for active office practice. But in order to do that he had to operate fast. Speed was paramount and a gastrectomy usually was completed in 90 minutes, skin to skin. He had his own nurse and first assistant, and the resident learned by watching.

I rotated on the service of another famous surgeon (we'll call him Dr. Pearl). He had a busy practice and operated on one of the giant Hollywood moguls, who offered him anything he wanted to come and play the part of a doctor in one of his movies. Pearl really looked the part. He was six-foot-two in height and somewhat bulky. He always wore a finely tailored pearl gray three-piece suit and had a diamond stickpin. His specialty was the six-minute cholecystectomy and 45-minute mastectomy.

Few patients had this latter operation without considerable blood loss. I hated the operation, until I eventually learned to do it without any blood loss when I was at the University of California. I subsequently became a noted breast surgeon in my own right, and never had to transfuse a patient of my own for this procedure in 35 years.

A few patients developed peritonitis after a gallbladder operation, and I thought for a while that this complication could occur easily in some of these cases. It wasn't until I got to California that I learned that careful surgery might take a bit longer. But there were no or rare complications. In those days there seemed to be a rivalry to see who could set a new speed record, or do the most cases in a week.

Once, when I covered Dr. Gross' cases at night, a patient started bleeding internally post-op. The leading surgeons all had "schleppers," young surgeons who got paid for assisting at operations and covering them on nights and weekends, so the older surgeons wouldn't have to come in to see emergencies. I suppose these young guys all hoped that some of the practice might rub off to them. One of these fellows came in and I told him we had trouble. A patient had post-operative bleeding. He was petrified that he might have to call his boss and refused until I threatened to take the patient back to the OR myself (which, of course, I couldn't do).

The old guy finally came in and we got the problem resolved in the OR with Dr. Gross cursing every step of the way. It was sometimes the job of the schleppers to take the blame for any mishap.

Dr. Pearl once admitted a world-famous economist and stock broker for a cholecystic-tomy. This was a man known throughout the financial world who had written several books. Post-op, I approached his bed. He was recovering well and I was pretty gutsy then. I passed a few pleasantries and made sure all was okay by examining his chest and abdomen. Then I asked him the key question: "How do you make money in the stock market?" I couldn't let this opportunity pass. He looked directly into my eyes and said, "That's easy, you buy and sell for other people." I never followed his advice, and was not very successful in the market either until much later in life.

Once a Hasidic pair of brothers came to Sinai after a four-hour trek from upstate New York—someplace in Sullivan County. There was never a thought of going anywhere else. This was the place for orthodox Jews to be treated. One had brought the other, who had a perforated appendix. He was pretty sick. The healthy one approached me and said he wanted Dr. Gross to do the operation. How much did I think it would cost?

I answered that I really didn't have any idea but I was sure it would be over $1,000. Actually, Dr. Gross rarely operated for less than $3,000. (This was 1957). The old man looked at me and said: "Maybe you shouldn't say anything to my brother."

I was assigned to the case, and I removed the appendix and he did fine. I suppose to this day he points to the scar with pride as the time Dr. Gross did his operation.

I was on another service when a surgeon scheduled a gastrectomy on a young woman. It was on the day I went to Washington to get my Air Force assignment. One of the other residents covered for me. The anastomosis leaked and she became deathly ill. After several days, Dr. Pearl was called in consultation but he didn't recommend any other treatment. Taking the patient back to the OR was not considered. I don't ever remember a mortality and morbidity conference to discuss complications as are now required by the surgical training review committees. I practically lived with that patient for the next two weeks, regulating her IVs and antibiotics, using every trick I could find in the literature, including using pooled gamma globulin. She eventually survived, to everyone's surprise and my relief.

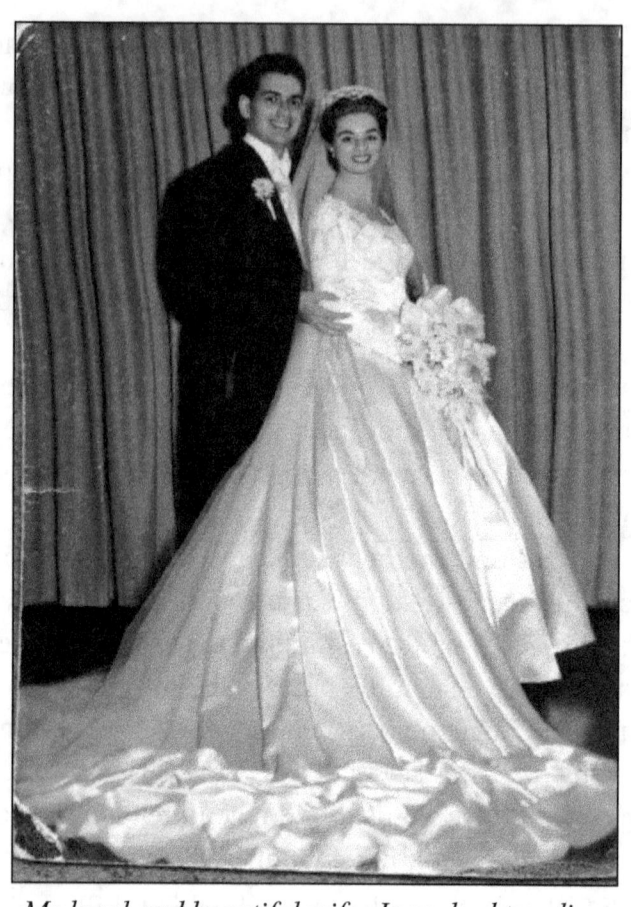

My loyal and beautiful wife, Joan, had to adjust to my hectic schedule as a young doctor.

My experiences at this hospital taught me an important lesson that has persisted, and a lesson that unfortunately most lay persons never appreciate. No matter how great a hospital's reputation is, you had better select the right doctor. Even later on, as I will relate, when I became chief of surgery at a large suburban hospital, this truism was driven home to me on many occasions. Most hospitals today can provide safe and efficient care, but there is a huge variation in the quality and motivations of the individual doctors on staff.

Joan learned early on that as a surgeon, I always believed that my patient's health took precedence over everything else. We celebrated New Year's Eve at the hospital with a party thrown by the resident staff. I wasn't on call, but one of my patients had to be taken back to the OR, and off I went with the patient. I was on the ward service at the time and we were responsible for our own patients. I don't remember the circumstances, except that Joan had to find her way home late at night by herself. All the years we were married she never complained once about anything I had to do that was necessary for my patients, even missing important events for the kids, or missing out on a Broadway play for which she had bought tickets months earlier. The patient did fine.

Occasionally a co-resident unfortunately got involved in a romantic encounter. I saw this again at Downstate when I was a faculty member, and some of my residents got into serious trouble. The divorce rate is pretty high among those residents who either can't avoid these liaisons or whose spouses never accommodate to the many hours spent at the hospital. By the way, some indiscretions also involve attending surgeons with nurses, and female residents with male residents.

My chief of surgery was an academic cardiac surgeon who ran into constant trouble with the famous practitioners at the hospital. This scenario will be described from my personal experience later. He tried to instill some science into the management of patients, a method that is standard in many institutions, but ran into a group of headstrong dilettantes that all had much more experience than he possessed. How do you teach a resident the proper approach to removing a colon for cancer when the private surgeon has been doing it in over a thousand cases his own way (and may not be using good cancer technique, in my opinion)? Experience is valuable, but surgeons tend to repress their bad results and promote their good results, which is undoubtedly a normal human response. But unless you subject the results to critical review, you cannot be certain that you are not repeating the same mistake each time. In private practice it was routine to refer the patients back to their family doctor for follow-up. As a result, many cancer patients may not have been adequately followed. As a rule I, or a medical oncologist, always followed my cancer patients, a practice that cost me many referrals. Nevertheless, our chief became more and more frustrated and more disorderly as a result of constant criticism and derision by the private guys.

One time, he asked a friend who was a leading academic surgeon, world famous for his work on ulcerative colitis, to give our grand rounds. After his presentation, he was asked by Dr. Gross how many colectomies he had done to reach his conclusions.

"About 125 over ten years," he responded.

"Well, I've removed over 1,200 colons and I don't agree with anything you've presented," was the response. I subsequently learned that our visiting professor was absolutely correct in many of his statements. Much of the progress in the treatment of this disease was made in other institutions by critical investigators.

Not that critical investigation wasn't going on at the hospital. It was in many areas, but except for one or two surgeons, usually outside of the surgery department. My chief, of course, didn't have the ears of the board which approved policy for the hospital, since the old-time surgeons had the reputation and had operated upon many of the board members or their families. It was easy to undermine his authority, and while I was in the military service my chief was fired. This, of course, put my future job in jeopardy and convinced us to try to stay in California, which we were thinking about anyhow. So on we went to UC San Francisco.

A word about technique. In later years I worked with a very busy medical oncologist. My usual colectomy included a careful removal of the node bearing mesentery of the involved segment, necessitating removal of a longer segment of colon. It added extra time to the procedure. Colon cancer is a rapidly growing cancer that metastasizes by invading lymph nodes, blood vessels or neighboring tissues. It often stays local for lengthy periods and thus can still be cured by an extended resection, even including nearby directly invaded organs, which I performed on multiple occasions. On occasion, I was able to cure patients with locally recurrent colon cancer and many surgeons have cured patients with liver metastases by resection.

One day, this oncologist told me that the colon cases I referred did very well and had fewer recurrences than his other referrals. He didn't understand the reason. A quick segmental resection was not my way.

Again, long hours were the mainstay of training. We had an easier time than previously, because the laboratories worked well and the blood bank was first class. The experiences on the private services were invaluable for caring for large numbers of operative cases under supervision. On the ward services, attending coverage was infrequent but available for very sick patients. The chief residents were responsible for patient care and no decisions were made without their acquiescence. They also decided who would operate on ward (non-private) patients and if a chief resident was "hungry" (had done few cases), almost nothing got passed down for the younger residents.

Commentary

As residents, we spent many long hours at the patient's bedside and saw firsthand the results of our treatment. I can't say that no mistakes were made, but none life-threatening. Surgeons make hundreds of decisions daily, from ordering IVs, medications, reviewing x-rays and many times we learned that it was better to make a wrong decision than no decision. This sounds strange, but a perfect example is the decision to operate on acute appendicitis. We are wrong 10 to 15% of the time (before modern radiological tests were available), but a delay in diagnosis in an acute case can lead to serious complications for the patient, or even death. (I have seen many examples of this in patients where significant delay in obtaining adequate surgical consultation was at fault.) We remove a few normal appendices (an error in diagnosis) in difficult diagnostic cases to avoid the possibility of complications occurring.

Delay in diagnosis is one of the leading causes of successful malpractice suits. I wrote a chapter on malpractice in the ER for a book by and for lawyers and commented (tongue in cheek) that the way to avoid a malpractice judgment was to operate early on all ER admissions with abdominal pain. (See later comments on morbidity and mortality conferences.)

Although the surgical residency was responsible for significant sleep deprivation, the line of command to the chief resident (and now to the attending faculty surgeon) was designed to avoid serious management errors. The experience, however, was invaluable in providing my management skills and decision-making ability which served my patients well over the years.

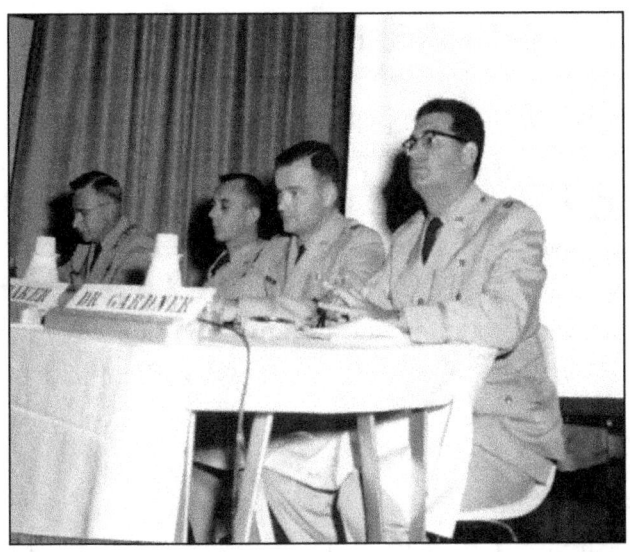

During my Air Force career, I joined in several symposia such as this one.

CHAPTER 3: IN THE AIR FORCE

I had a month of preliminary military training at Gunther Air Force Base in Montgomery, Alabama. This was cross-town from the home of the Air University at Maxwell Air Force Base, which had at least four generals on base. The Officer's Club looked like a dance floor from the Waldorf Astoria in New York. You were greeted by an officer in dress uniform and guided to your table. A live orchestra played various dance tunes and the food and service was outstanding. All for a few dollars.

An elderly officer and his spouse danced every dance, and regardless of the music they did a Peabody across the floor, in a glorious floatation to whatever rhythm the orchestra came up with. We deeply admired them. This was a great break from the dull lectures of the preceding afternoons.

We drove to California by way of Reno and signed in to Travis Air Force base.

I learned a few things about the military during my 23 months at Travis. Travis Air Force base was a MATS Base (military air transport), which was responsible for carrying personnel and equipment all over the world. Planes took off regularly from Travis to all points in the Far East, carrying people going on assignment or returning home. There was a large hospital on base, which served as a local hospital for the large number of personnel and families on base, as a regional referral center covering several western states, and as a center for determining discharge disabilities. There was a SAC unit also assigned to Travis. This was the famous Strategic Air Command, which was our retaliatory arm in the event of a nuclear attack. Planes from several of these units from various bases were in the air at all times so as not to have the long-range bombers caught on the ground at any one time.

At the time of my arrival, Travis was to take over the entire western region and Parks Air Force Base, a few miles away and also with a very large hospital, was scheduled to close. The way I got this choice assignment was interesting. I was deferred for two years during my internship and first year of residency, as I indicated previously, in order to qualify for a surgical rating. I had heard that if you went to Washington and asked for specific assignments you could get them. So off I went.

In the Pentagon, I was directed to a colonel in charge of assignments for medical officers in the Air force, and he took me to the Airman second class who really made all the decisions. This young man was a very pleasant fellow. I originally asked for assignment to Wiesbaden in Germany, but this required an additional year of service. I wasn't interested. I asked for the largest hospital available in a pleasant climate and was asked if the San Francisco area was okay. You bet it was! He stood in front of a large map of the world with a lot of pins, picked one up and stuck it in Travis AFB, and I was set for the next two years.

As I had mentioned, Parks Hospital was set to close for several years, and this was actually completed when I arrived at Travis. The last unit to leave the hospital were the nurses and doctors. As they arrived at Travis, I heard stories that a private company had just started to paint the walls of the hospital at Parks. Some efficiency!

When we arrived, we placed a call to our friend Stan Goldberg in Berkeley. The operator came on line and we said Goldberg. "How do you spell that?" she said. Welcome to California.

We lived in Wherry housing on base. We had a choice of living there or getting an allowance to live off-base in Fairfield. The convenience of being so close to work really thrilled this old New Yorker. The house was a single level ranch with three rooms and one bath. Pure luxury for us. You entered a small foyer and the kitchen was immediately to the left. There was a door that you opened to get to the kitchen and it didn't make much sense to walk into the house and have a closed door right near the entrance. I therefore filed a petition to have the door removed, and the immense number of forms were filled out by a helpful airman first class. Meanwhile I figured out a way of widely opening the door against a wall so that it didn't appear obtrusive.

We met the base commander on arrival and were given a lecture on how officers were expected to behave. He showed us the requisite shoe polish and brush in his lower desk drawer. Actually, the base was run by the non-commissioned officers who could get anything done. They had great respect for the doctors on base, who could guarantee immediate care for their families, and medications for sick kids without long delays at the hospital emergency room or clinic. This turned out to be a beautiful symbiotic relationship—except for my door.

The staff at the hospital consisted of regular Air Force docs whose main interest, it seemed, was in lining up at the door by four-thirty waiting for dismissal to sound. They then headed directly to the Officers' Club for happy hour. Then there were short-timers like me, who took care of the patients at all hours. We worked with the techs (who eventually developed into what we now know as physician assistants), who really did the bulk of the work. They started the IVs, scrubbed on the OR cases as first or second assistants, did all the paperwork, organized the clinics, wrote orders and almost never got anything wrong. I was there to oversee the care and do the hands-on patients work.

I was lucky to be assigned to surgery for my entire stay. Some of the other guys who arrived with me didn't fare as well. One fellow, a budding pathologist, ended up as a pediatrician. An OB-GYN-trained surgeon became the new pathologist. The Air Force figured that as long as you had that MD after your name, you could do anything in the medical field. This philosophy led to some interesting assignments on the smaller bases.

At Travis this didn't matter as much, because we had specialists who completed their residency training under the Berry Plan and owed time (usually at least five years) to the military. These were the fully trained doctors. By the time they had paid back this time they had ten years in, and it didn't take much more to stay for twenty and retire on a pension. Some of these doctors were really good and could teach me a lot in the OR. We had a fully trained cardiothoracic surgeon and did some open-heart procedures at the early development of this field. So, to review: there were three levels of specialty care: D level specialists (like me) who had 1 year of specialty residency (2 years of surgical training including the internship); full residency trained (board eligible) specialists, paying back time; and career medical officers.

One of our full timers (career officers) had trained at a famous clinic in the Midwest. He was a balding gentleman who just wasn't looking to operate. He outranked all of us. With a great deal of care, we usually managed to assign the simpler cases to him as well as most of the paper work. He didn't mind as long as he got to the officers' club by five o'clock.

Drinking was a major activity on base. The pilots who returned from Japan usually had orders for gallon bottles of scotch, which for them was duty free. Joan and I learned about this pretty quickly. As we were moving in, one of our neighbors dropped by to help. We had a couple of bottles half-full of scotch and gin, which we nursed for company over the years. By the time we had our barrels emptied, so were the bottles of booze. Needless to say, we were on the next list of goods from Japan. But liquor was cheap at the clubs. Fifty cents a drink and half price at happy hour. There was an AA group on the base, and at the front entrance of the base was a wrecked car as a reminder of the rewards of driving drunk. But as far as I could see, that didn't slow down the enormous alcohol consumption.

Our furniture was pretty sparse and arrived with the usual breakage and scratches. We didn't have one bit of trouble with claims, however, since the van lines we used weren't about to antagonize the non-coms on base. These fellows were in the position of referring all sorts of business, since much of the personnel were constantly moving to or off the base. The movers went to extremes to avoid complaints, particularly from the medical officers.

Each day at the hospital, we noticed a group of engineers walking around with notebooks and pencils. It seemed they decided we needed another elevator and were developing plans for this. For my entire stay they dug into the walls and finally constructed a shaft for the elevator. It was a mess. On the final day, after two years of construction, when the elevator was scheduled to start running, someone took out the plans of the hospital and discovered that an elevator shaft was already in place just around the corner from the newly constructed one. Somebody opened a door to the shaft early on, got a rush of air in their face and decided that the shaft was part of the air-conditioning system.

It was hard to outsmart the military. Our radiologist figured that there were so many routine chest x-rays taken, all of which had the same reading, that it would save a lot of time to make up a stamp which described a normal chest x-ray. So in went the usual requisitions and sixteen months later the appropriate stamp arrived—but with the signature and title of the radiologist he had replaced. It seems that gentleman had the same idea.

But not everything took so long to requisition. This same radiologist had developed a system of filing reports in manila folders and figured he needed about 100,000 to last for his two-year stint. Reckoning with the usual military mentality he ordered 250,000 (usually you're lucky to get half of what you ask for). Well, I suppose that someone was absolutely ecstatic when they got this request. Pretty soon 500,000 manila folders arrived.

They clogged up the x-ray department for months, with everyone tripping over cartons filled with manila folders.

They often had entertainment at the officers' club with a singer and a dance band. We had our own circle of friends usually. But soon after we just arrived we heard that a comedian was going to perform. We made reservations for ourselves and went since we hadn't met too many people as yet. Well I can't remember the comedian's name, but he was terrific. I don't usually laugh out loud. For me a smirk means that something is funny and a smile means it's hilarious. Well, this guy started telling jokes about the garment center in New York and both Joan and I were in the aisles. I think we were embarrassing ourselves with giant guffaws with each of his stories. But nobody else even smiled. The comedian was dead in his tracks. This was a rude introduction to life outside of the big city. I must say that this poor guy owed something to the agent that booked him into this deadpan audience.

We made a lot of friends during our stay, mostly short timers like us. There were two neurologists and a neurosurgeon on base, since we had to evaluate all of the regular Air Force personnel who claimed injuries for disability pensions. When you retired with a pension after 20 or 30 years, any percentage disability you could claim would make that part of your pension tax-free. There were other benefits, including VA care for the rest of your life. Since you couldn't deny somebody a pension who complained of work-related back pain, this was the most common complaint. Thus all these neurological specialists. A full and complete evaluation included a myelogram, and our neurosurgeon figured anyone sturdy (or stupid) enough to risk one of those tests probably had real back pain. Anyhow, this was a standard and popular method of completing your military stay. Everyone came out with a disability rating. We didn't have MRIs then, and most of the diagnoses of disc disease were based on a good history. Needless to say, many of those coming through had a well-rehearsed story to tell.

The neurologists were highly trained, from important New York programs, and eventually returned there in teaching capacities. They had the usual mistrust of surgeons. One of them carried a little note in a shirt pocket that read: "If I fall out of bed and am unconscious, call a neurologist, not a neurosurgeon."

One day the base commander, a two-star general, got a headache. Our internist called one of the neurologists. This poor fellow thought that he had an incurable brain tumor and underwent many neurological tests. After about three weeks of workup, the general was informed that he was going to live. They then cured the headache with treatment for a clogged frontal sinus. About a month later the neurologists got TDY (temporary duty with full pay and all travel paid for) orders to travel around the world to various air bases. They took off immediately and made the trip about two days ahead of orders canceling it. It pays to know the right general.

Travel in the Air Force can be a pleasant (although often frustrating) experience. Airplanes are always taking off and going someplace, and if you can hitch a ride you can get anywhere. Pilots or flight surgeons are required to maintain a certain amount of air time and are usually willing to take you on a trip. If the pilot is heading in a similar direction you can hitch rides to eventually get to where you want by hitching rides at bases along the way. I took a trip home by way of three air force bases over a two-day period. Since it's all free, many officers take advantage of this. "If you've got time to spare, go by air" is the motto.

In addition to this method, many military are always traveling to places on leave or with transfer orders or home. The military never had enough aircraft for all of these trips, and therefore arranged for civilian carriers to take these passengers on a space available basis. Since we were on a large base as a takeoff point for the Far East, many commercial carriers carrying a light load of passengers would land to pick up space available people. They of course got paid for this. Most travelers on base stayed in the barracks waiting for an appropriate flight to land, which could take a number of days. They were then notified to high- tail it over to the airfield when the plane was available.

Joan and I decided to take a vacation in Hawaii. We had a significant advantage since we lived on base. I had taken care of a non-com who knew the flight controller, and we would be notified when a flight to Hawaii had space. This meant I didn't have to sign out until we were ready to take off. We got the call, I drove over to hospital and signed out, returned to pick up Joan and the luggage, and we were off. The airline we got assigned to was a small carrier consisting of two planes. Apparently the owner told the Air Force he wanted to fly people to the Pacific and they said okay. I imagined that with that promise, he borrowed money from a bank and bought two old airplanes. With the airplanes in hand, he went back to the Air Force and got a contract to fly space available. He was in business.

The airline was really low-budget. The stewardess's uniforms consisted of a clean white blouse and a dark skirt. We took off and were well onto the Pacific when I looked out of the window and noticed that one of our starboard engines was on fire. At that moment, the captain was passing us on the way to the toilet. I stopped him, pointed to the engine and said, "I think something's wrong."

"Yeah, you're right" he answered, and went back and turned the engine off. We made the rest of the trip to Hawaii on three engines. This really must have been low-budget. The plane continued to Guam after dropping us off at Hickam Air Force Base. After our week in Hawaii, we again got space available and guess what. We had the same plane and crew going back, and surprise, they still hadn't fixed the engine. It made the entire trip out and back on three engines. (I don't think we would do that today.) I later heard a rumor that they went out of business when they couldn't get credit to buy gasoline at the airfields.

I'm not going to say much about Hawaii except that the trip was great.

We still didn't have much money, and being able to stay at Fort DeRussy, which had the best stretch of beach on Waikiki, for $1.50 a night was a gift for us. Drinks at the next-door Hawaiian Village were

$4 apiece, pretty expensive in those days, so we had a pre-dinner cocktail at our officers' club for fifty cents. The accommodations were not outstanding, but we had our own room, with a communal bathroom. However, the major disadvantage were huge numbers of roaches which roamed the halls at night. It was important to take care of all your needs before retiring. Well, what do you expect for a buck fifty?

Hawaii was sold as paradise, and every street corner with a view of anything was labeled a Kodak spot. We did all the things that tourists do, including going to a luau. I read the menu the day before and was very apprehensive about the raw fish we were going to eat. (No sushi in those days!) When I tasted it, something seemed familiar. Then I realized I had been eating raw fish for years. It tasted like herring in wine —and it probably was.

We took a fishing trip while on the island. Joan got seasick and did the usual thing. We didn't know then that she was finally pregnant. None of the other couples on board (there were two others) were interested in returning to port. Poor Joan toughed it out, as she did for many other situations in our future.

We bought a dog while we were in the service. Actually, we got it for nothing from the pound. It was mostly a cocker spaniel, tan and we named him

Brandy. Although lovable, he was incredibly stupid. He loved to ride in the car, and many times to appease him, we'd let him into the car and after a few minutes let him out. He thought he'd been driving for hours. He had a few problems, however. The main one was that he hated people in uniform, pretty tough when you live on base. In addition, he had a special greeting for new friends, which consisted of sidling over and urinating on their shoes. Other than those few faults, he was an adorable pet.

You might think it was tough living on base, with planes taking off all the time. Actually, you get used to it. By the middle of the month the number of takeoffs seemed to decrease, and by the end of the month there were hardly any. I surmised that the budget was assigned in monthly allotments, and the worst sin was to have money left over at the month's end. To avoid this, all money was spent at the beginning of each month, and by the end the gas was pretty well used up. I thought we were lucky that the Russians didn't attack us on the thirtieth of the month. I wasn't sure we'd be able to retaliate.

A few words about the mentality of the regular officers. I remember an episode at the officers' club when a pilot was publicly reprimanded for not taking off with his unit that morning. He responded that his plane had serious engine trouble and wouldn't start. It didn't matter, screamed his commanding officer, it was his job to take off (SAC) and no excuses would be tolerated.

We had one adjutant on the base who was in charge of cleanup and the appearance of the base. He gave himself a ticket for not mowing his own lawn.

About eight months into my stay, we had a visit from an airman who came to look at my door to the kitchen. He looked at it right and left and casually strolled around it. I asked him what he was doing and he responded that he had to file a report to the committee indicating how many personnel it would take to remove the door.

A few months before we left the base, another airman arrived the house. We had completely adjusted to the fact that the door was there to stay. He came, and with a retractable tape measured the height, width, thickness and anything else he could of that door. His response to my usual query was that he had to file a report as to how much storage space the door would take up after it was removed. You'd think that somewhere, someone would know the size of a standard Wherry door.

Well, clearly they were still holding meetings about my door. I was sure that when the next couple moved in, the door would be off and they would spend two years trying to get it put back on.

It wouldn't be right to skip over the medical aspects of military life. This was as close to socialized medicine as you could get in America. Everything was covered and paid for. The clinics and emergency services were always busy. Women who had little to do would think nothing of meeting their friends at the hospital and get checked over for some complaint. It was often more social than medical. This was the only time in my career that I saw patients with abdominal pain of 10 minutes duration.

This was quite different from my days at the charity hospital where patients came to the hospital as a last resort—usually after a major complication had occurred.

If you needed a heart operation, or had a major burn, or a perforated ulcer, the treatment you got was superb. If you had a headache, you got very superficial treatment, and in fact with many complaints an occasional major catastrophe was missed.

This was of course due to the large number of visits of patients with trivial symptoms.

I want to stress that my observations all pertain to a peacetime situation. During wartime, many of the doctors and surgeons who retained reserve status return to active duty. The accomplishments of these physicians are amazing for the large number of lives saved under the most trying conditions. I would give kudos to the military airmen and doctors who put their lives on the line many times.

In addition, my knowledge and experience with treatment and rehabilitation at VA hospitals indicates they are the best in the world.

We left the Air Force much richer than we arrived. We had adopted a little newborn girl, and Joan was finally pregnant with our second daughter. We decided to stay in California, as my former chief had been fired at Mt. Sinai. I arranged a fellowship at The University of California in San Francisco and was to enter the surgical residency program the following year. The fellowship paid a living wage, and I was going to make $170 a month after that, with all meals paid for and an allowance for housing. We could make it with a loan from my brother-in-law, with which we bought an inexpensive house on the San Andreas Fault. This was ours for the next five years.

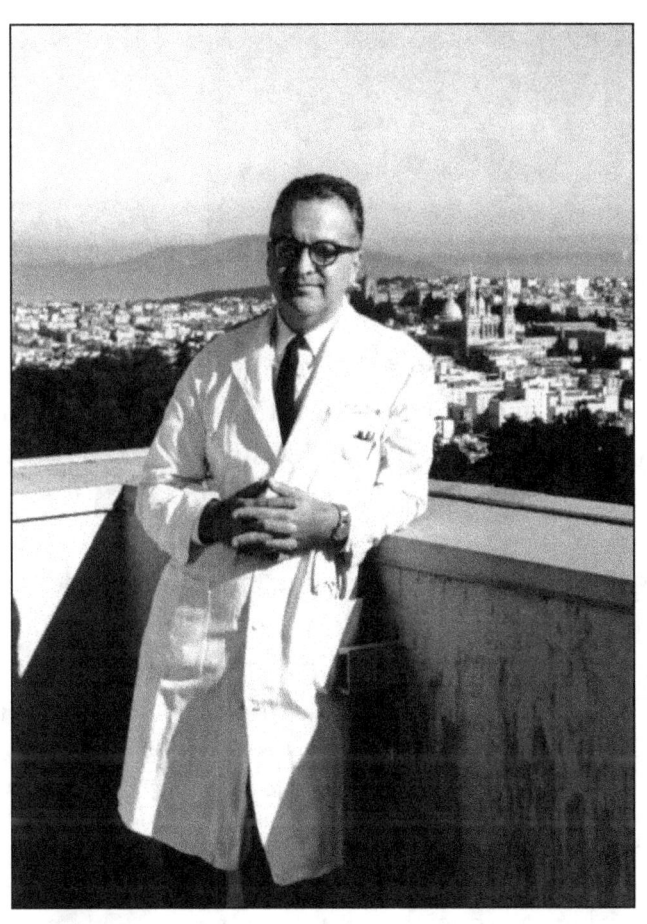

CHAPTER 4: AT CALIFORNIA

The University of California at San Francisco is and was one of the most prestigious institutions for surgical training in the country. In order to be accepted into the program I had to take a year of research, which turned out to be one of the best years of the whole training program. I had my introduction to patients with breast cancer, and actually published eight papers during that year. This was in addition to making presentations at a number of important medical meetings.

I worked under the tutelage of a brilliant investigator, Gil Gordan. He could quote articles from the medical literature of thirty years ago as quickly as one he read yesterday. On many occasions he would give me the exact journal and page reference of a paper to solve a problem I was having in the lab. I don't remember him ever being wrong. He was also a generous and supportive man to all that worked with him. He was a good and close friend with a wide variety of interests. It was not a problem for him to learn Spanish in order to give a paper in South America. He loved to grow orchids and was a connoisseur of wines and brandies from all over the world. He spoke a number of languages and was at home anywhere in the world that his research took him, a true Renaissance man. He was an endocrinologist, and in those days the endocrinologists treated advanced breast cancer, since no chemotherapy was as yet proven to be effective in this disease.

We had a clinic of over 100 patients in all stages of breast cancer, which gave me the opportunity to study calcium metabolism, renal dynamics (kidney function), and metastases in this disease. I learned to use hormones and to follow patients after adrenalectomy or hypophysectomy. We had many long survivors.

Like many surgical residents in a laboratory, I was very productive and put in many hours of extra time. This still was a vacation compared to what was to follow. We became personally friendly with Gil, his secretary and her family, and the families of many of his lab aides. On many occasions we were invited to cocktail or dinner parties at his home and met many famous and distinguished researchers from all parts of the world. These men and women came to pay homage to Gil, and to review work that they had in common.

What was most surprising was the respect Gil had for his lab technicians, Ph.D. candidates and secretaries. We were all treated like family and spent many evenings together at one or another's home. This was so different from the atmosphere I experienced back east, where it was rare for bosses and their research assistants to socialize. Gil took a genuine interest in our personal problems, and it was natural for me to ask him to be godfather to our son.

I remember having the Gordans and staff over for dinner, and Joan made a dish called country captain chicken, which took two days to prepare. Everyone was complimentary and seemed to enjoy the dish, and as they left, Gil's wife whispered to me "Gil never ate chicken—until tonight."

Most of all, Gil loved San Francisco. He lived on Twin Peaks, that area that provides a magnificent view of the city, Golden Gate Bridge and also the East Bay. And we learned to love San Francisco as well.

But the Bay Area has one major problem—FOG. We were two blocks from the ocean and almost never saw the sun. That is Joan and the kids didn't. I worked on Mt. Parnassus, where the fog broke, and had beautiful weather. I dreaded calling home and having to tell Joan that it was another sunny day in town. I never used a topcoat in the seven years we lived in the Bay Area (and Travis), but the kids needed warm jackets to make it through the summer in Westlake.

San Francisco is known as the air-conditioned city due to the fog. It usually peters out over the Twin Peaks area, leaving most of the downtown area sunny by late morning. Most visitors don't realize the problems, but if you're going to buy a home, you'd better know where the fog belts are in town.

We spent my occasional weekends off driving out of Westlake to the sun, south of San Bruno or into Marin County. We peeled off the layers of clothing down to bathing suits and had a picnic in a number of public parks in these areas. Aside from the fog, the Bay Area and peninsula is the greatest place in the country to live, both from the point of the best climate and beauty of the coast and cliffs along the shore. Those mountains are now covered with homes and developments and the entire area south to San Jose along the coast seems like one city.

When visitors and family came, we took them on drives through town and into the surrounding wine country. We'd stop at a village market on the way and pick up some bread and cheese, and then head for the wine tasting rooms in Napa Valley. One time while we were savoring some wine with friends, a lady came over to our table and accused us of hogging the bread and cheese. I guess she thought the wineries provided lunch also.

I have to say some things about surgical residencies. When I got back to a formal residency,

I didn't see my family regularly. In the program we rotated between the University Hospital and San Francisco General. At both institutions we were on duty 365 days and nights per year. Any time off, including vacations, was arranged by getting coverage from a resident at the same level of training. We were permitted to take calls from home, but because of the load of patients we managed, seldom had the chance. Looking back on those years, I would have to say that I really learned a lot, and the training was superb. For many years I would never answer a phone at home if anyone else was around, because it was always associated in my mind with a major problem of some sort.

I often tell students who need guidance in selecting a career to make certain if they choose surgery that they marry someone who is willing to accept your total commitment to your patients. I thank heaven that I made the right choice.

Surgical residencies are X-rated. Not because of sexual experiences but because of the injuries, blood and wounds with which you have to deal. San Francisco is the suicide capital of the world, and we saw plenty of those. A particularly tough one was a man who put a shotgun to his chin, fired and missed everything vital. Except he had no face when he arrived in the ER.

We had to resuscitate him and plan his treatment and rehabilitation over the hospitalization. He didn't want to live and did eventually die after a number of months from a lung infection.

We had the largest hand clinic in the country dealing with wrist lacerations. We would repair these and follow the patients for years, watching and recording every improvement in motion of the fingers, documenting our results. These operations would take six or seven hours to perform. Often, after years of rehabilitation, some of these patients would show up in the ER again having slashed their wrists a second time.

One night, we were notified of a major accident on the Bay Bridge. A drunken driver had jumped the divider and hit oncoming cars. I notified my chief resident and he hurried down to the ER. He admitted his parents, who were among the victims. His father couldn't be saved, but he resuscitated and operated on his mother who survived, although with major disabilities.

We had two surgical services and two sister medical services at the general hospital. We were on call one week straight and off the following week for night call. The problem was that our medical service, which admitted with us, usually had a flock of patients ready for the OR on the week we had nights off. Essentially, we didn't get home too often. I remember one specific weekend when I was chief resident, and we admitted 23 patients. We slept in two- or three-hour shifts (there were four of us on call) so we could rotate in the OR. By the time an acute appendicitis rolled in on Monday morning, we were pretty giddy and could only stand and laugh. This doesn't happen anymore, as resident duty hours are strictly limited.

In spite of the long hours, we were dedicated to our surgical education. As chief resident, I often arranged with the anatomy department for a cadaver to be available on a Sunday (a day off for some of us), so we could dissect some area of interest. Four or five residents would work together to improve our recognition of anatomical nuances that could help us in the OR.

One day a week, we started our evening rounds in the pathology department, so we could review the previous week's specimens and slides. In this way we had the opportunity to see, under the microscope, the tissues we had removed. This provided knowledge that was useful in later years, when we looked at frozen sections of tissues excised at operation in order to determine how to proceed. I don't ever recall any of my residents complaining that he or she would rather be at home sleeping than participate in these teaching exercises. They usually asked for more.

San Francisco is a city that attracts young women from all over the country, and unfortunately not an equal number of young men. With a large population of gay men, the women severely outnumber possible matches. Therefore nothing is sacred in trying to get a date. Many of the single nurses try to find doctors (or residents), and it often doesn't matter if they are married. After all, who knows what trouble a marriage might be in? I was invited to dinner by a lovely young nurse from the surgical ICU who was uncomfortably attentive. I decided to bring Joan along, pretending that the invitation was for both of us. Needless to say this was an awkward and very strange evening, even though there were two other couples present.

The spaghetti and meatballs were delicious, but the conversation was a bit sparse. This, however, put to rest any additional attention I might have received during the remainder of my residency.

My rotations at the University Hospital were not quite as hectic as they were at the General, but we were never officially off-call. On the private service, we scrubbed with a variety of surgeons. As opposed to the atmosphere in my previous years, which was directed at how fast the operation could be done, at Cal the procedures were carefully performed and the stress was on avoiding complications. Good surgical technique was the key, and I learned its importance during this period of time. For the first time, I saw breast and gallbladder surgery performed which never required a blood transfusion, and after which the patients recovered promptly and were discharged early. The techniques I developed there have always done well for me and my patients, and helped me to train a large number of surgical residents.

As residents, we were not privy to the infighting, which I'm sure existed, and which affects much of medical practice, but I will get to those aspects later. However, there was a distinct difference in the cooperation between the medical and surgical services as compared to my previous experience. As a chief resident, I was frequently asked to make rounds on the medical service with their residents, and on many occasions was asked for management opinions which may have included an operation as one choice. There was no attempt to hide patients, and on some occasions patients were transferred between the services for better management.

When I subsequently left Downstate as a professor, years later, one of the parties for me was given by friends on the medical service. I would, however, make one caveat. On many occasions, the medical interns were left to themselves to manage very complicated cases at night. Medical resident coverage was poor at the county hospital. There didn't seem to be the control or graded responsibility that was ingrained in, surgical residencies. This was my limited observation and may not reflect other programs or subsequent changes.

Seven months after adopting our beautiful little daughter at Travis, Joan gave birth to another beautiful daughter. These were like twins and were brought up that way. With two little ones and very little money, Joan sought help from her mother, who flew out from New York. She picked up one of the babies and hurt her back. Joan now had three to take care of. As I noted before, I was of little help.

It amazes me how far our salary went in those days. We saved money from our Air Force days and managed very well. The girls had clothing to wear, and we ate out once a week and paid a mortgage to boot. We had a large group of friends and friendly neighbors, all young couples with children. Needless to say, living in the fog, on the fault, was inexpensive.

My chief of surgery at Cal was a compassionate and excellent surgeon. The University medical school was gradually being converted from a center

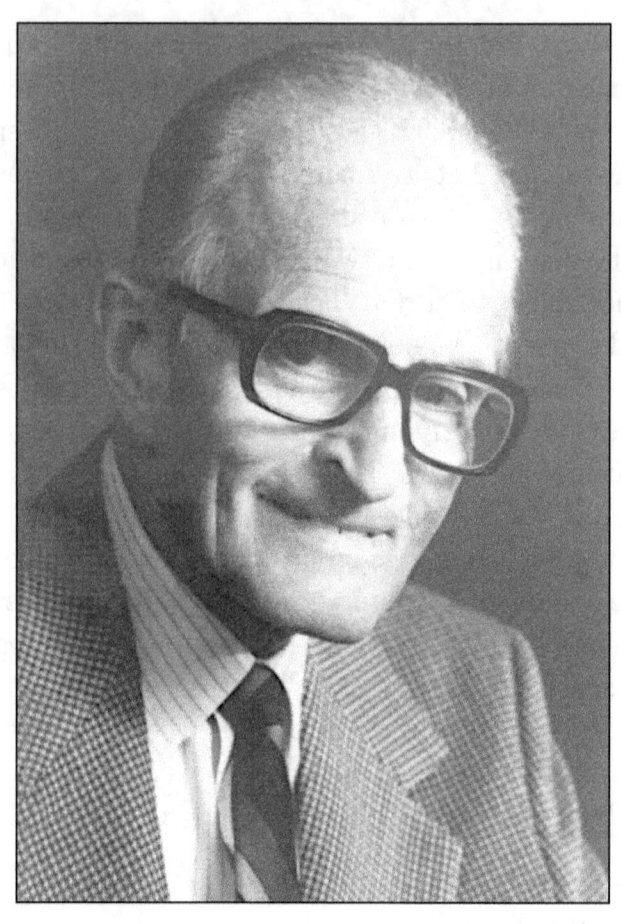

Leon Goldman, was chief of surgery during my stay at Cal.

of private practice to an academic center. Research was not a prime factor for faculty when the institution first developed, and in the late 1950s and early '60s these attitudes were changing. Our chief, Leon Goldman, was a transition to this new attitude. He developed the concept of sending bright young members of the surgical faculty to the laboratories of famous researchers and then bringing them back as faculty to start research programs within the department. Some of these surgeons went on to great fame and became leaders of their own departments at Harvard and Minnesota, among other places.

But one tradition did not change, and that was that the residents on the ward services had the primary responsibility for the care of the patients. These patients were referred to the institution, rather than specific surgeons, or referred themselves to clinics when they couldn't pay the private surgical fees. While an attending surgeon saw and was informed of the developments, the resident usually operated without direct supervision. The theory was that you became a chief resident when you were ready for this responsibility. We were ready, and I looked forward to doing these cases. But I have to admit that there were times I wish we had an attending surgeon in the room with us. It hurts to review some of these cases, particularly an occasional patient who had a very complicated problem. This doesn't exist much today in most programs.

When I joined the faculty at Downstate and subsequently, I always scrubbed with the residents, frequently until the dressing was on, even though they thought that they were doing the case. When I was in charge of a large service, I set up a system of having the faculty responsible for seeing patients preoperatively and scrubbing on every case. The residents were usually grateful. It certainly cut down on operating time.

Interestingly, we did a study comparing results of attending and resident cases and there were no differences in complication rates between the groups. This was undoubtedly due to the large volume of cases we scrubbed on at Cal, a condition not available at most institutions today.

There are certainly some institutions today where the house staff are poorly supervised. These situations always involve patients that are indigent or uninsured. Anyone who doubts that, in large segments of our medical world, a double standard of care exists has probably got sand coming out of his ears. Interestingly, some of the institutions that function this way are among the most well known in the country. Many are in large cities and have large private patient clientele, but even some of these patients with poor insurance, are left for the residents to manage.

Rural areas may have difficulties in attracting highly trained specialists. Hospitals may be long distances from patients. Trauma treatment is closely monitored in some states and air transport is provided to level one facilities. But patients requiring special expertise may not have it easily available, unless they can afford to pay for transportation to a specialty hospital. In some cases, it is cheaper for patients to leave the country for operations they cannot afford in the U.S. We are the only civilized country which does not guarantee health care to its citizens.

Additionally: many friends and relatives have asked for advice on choosing medical care. I always insist on the following. Look for a doctor who will give devoted attention to your problem and has the expertise to handle it, and most importantly, recognizes his own limitations. He should have no qualms about bringing in a consultant if the family requests one or if he needs help. It makes no difference if he or she is on the staff of a large university hospital or large voluntary community teaching hospital. Never choose a hospital without knowing precisely which doctor you will see. (see Chapter 9)

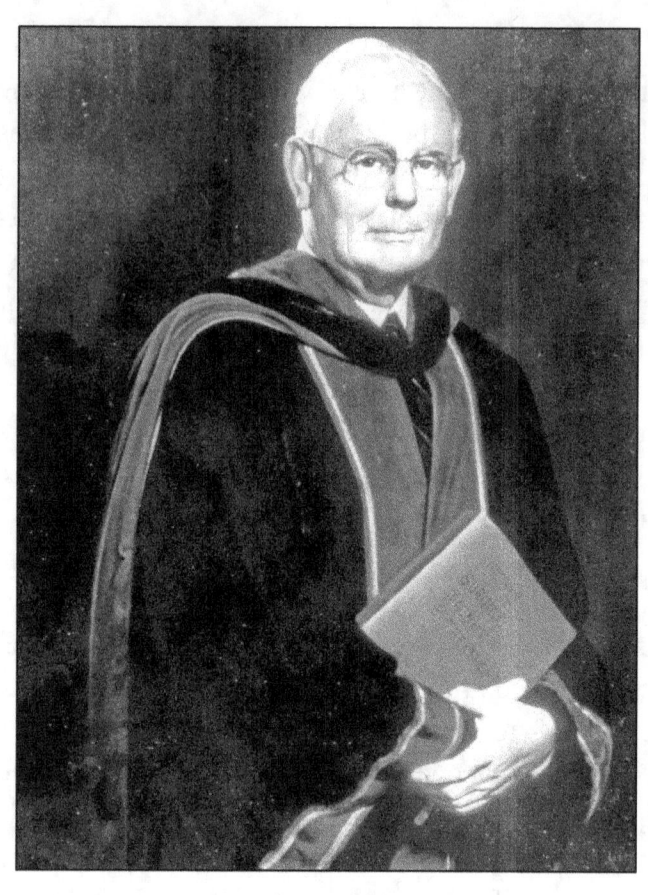

J. Englebert Dunphy

I spent five years at Cal. In my chief resident year, we got a new chief of surgery, J. Englebert Dunphy. This was a little Irishman who was world-famous as a surgeon, and a researcher and especially as a teacher. He had been president of almost every prestigious surgical society. He established rules so that every complication or mortality was discussed in detail and assistant residents had to report these so that the chief residents or attendings would not be tempted to cover anything up. (I later tried this at a community hospital and was severely taken to task.) He had a wonderful sense of humor and the knack of making you laugh, even when you were being severely criticized. Surgeons came from all over San Francisco to attend these sessions. If you did things his way, you got along fine.

We had superb residents at Cal in those days. One of the best was an assistant resident named, we'll say, Jones. One day, Dr. Dunphy called me into his office. "I want you to fire Jones," he said.

Stunned I reiterated that Jones was doing his usual excellent job.

"I don't care," Dunphy said, "I got a call from the record room that Jones hasn't signed out his charts, and I haven't got the time to deal with this kind of problem." Well, with much cajoling on my part, we agreed that the charts would be completed promptly and Jones could keep his job. Of course, Dunphy had no intention of firing this excellent resident—contrary to what happened at my first hospital—but was making a point. No resident had incomplete records for a long time once the word got around.

During my residency at Cal I continued some research with the help of Gil Gordan and ended up with about sixteen publications. I also did a huge number of operations, which were available in those days. In my chief year I completed almost 600 procedures. I was a pretty tough chief, and my residents were expected to work as hard as I did. Their first priority was to the patients. As my chief residents had taught me, I taught them how to operate and make decisions. To this day, there are many stories about my tenure still going on at Cal, and I maintain contact with many of my residents in academic surgery.

Joan and I were committed to returning to New York. We adopted a beautiful baby boy, and we both felt that it would be important for the three children to get to know their family, aunts, uncles, and cousins and grandparents. I felt I would continue in academic surgery and wrote letters to various institutions in the New York area. I didn't have much of a response from any of the Manhattan medical schools, in spite of my background in research. I did get a job offer from the State

University of New York, Downstate Medical School in Brooklyn and off we went. I might have stayed at Cal and some years later, when I had won the prestigious Markle Scholarship, I met Dunphy and he apologized for not offering me a job at Cal.

The coverage tradition for residents at Cal was the severest I had witnessed. We spent an enormous amount of time taking care of patients. The tradition at the county hospital was for the chief resident to have full responsibility. Attending coverage was sparse, and usually only available by phone. We would call and explain the case and review our planned treatment. The okay was given by the attending without his seeing the patient. We had better coverage at the University Hospital because there were few emergencies, and the attendings could see the patients' pre-op and schedule time to look in the OR or be present at the operation. Rounds were made regularly on both ward and private patients.

This is very different from today, when attending physicians often sleep at the hospital (required at all level 1 trauma centers) and are usually available for consultation night and day. Most residents do not have privileges to operate independently except on minor procedures, such as drainage of an abscess. Institutions vary in how residents are covered by attendings. At some, a super resident (one who has completed his or her residency) is given a faculty position to cover patients who are uninsured (formerly the ward service). They scrub with the residents on all cases, although they may not be experienced in the procedure at hand. At other institutions, attendings specialize in certain areas and will be called to assist the chief resident in those specific areas. From the resident's point of view, scrubbing with the more experienced surgeon is preferable.

Residents do not have the experience today that we had when I trained. I had already performed well over 1,000 supervised operations before I became chief resident. Even with assisting the younger residents in that year, I still personally performed over 600 major procedures in my chief year. At Cal, patients referred to the university without or with poor insurance became resident cases. Today, the experience is greatly limited by shorter, controlled work hours during the assistant residency, and therefore coverage by experienced attending surgeons is vital for adequate training and patient safety. Furthermore, as our trained residents and fellows go into private practice in the geographical area where they trained, fewer patients are referred to the university, leaving fewer resident cases.

Therefore, many surgical residents feel the need to go for additional training in specialty fellowships. Now, some leaders are considering an additional year in general surgery. This is detrimental to the residency, as it reduces even further the experience of residents in the program. It generally reflects the fact that there are too few cases for resident training or too many residents in the program, which most chairmen won't admit.

The Morbidity and Mortality Conference

Every complication of operations, or management of non-operative cases, is supposed to be discussed at a weekly conference including all attending physicians (staff), residents and often students. This is now a standard board requirement for program approval. This was done at Cal, Downstate, and New Jersey Medical School. These conferences generally provide a list of every operation by surgeon or service, and the chief selects those cases where long and detailed discussion may be fruitful as teaching points, or to prevent repeated errors. Anyone attending the conference may comment, and often the discussions may become heated. The final arbitrator is often the pertinent surgical literature, so that evidence-based opinions are most valued.

In the past, discussions held at these conferences were considered privileged and not subpoenable to avoid compromising the honest presentation of facts and opinions. Without this protection, most surgeons would be loath to have their cases presented. Data on infection rates and mortalities are also presented. Presentation doesn't depend on whether the complication was due to error or was expected. If done seriously, this conference remains a primary tool in reducing complication rates. Not all hospitals have such a conference.

As an example: we had a well-respected urologist introduce peritoneal lavage (as done for dialysis) post-operatively as a treatment in patients operated upon with ruptured bowel. The intent was to reduce bacterial contamination and improve survival in this group of patients, who usually had high mortality. After multiple consecutive deaths, I posed the question at a mortality conference that we may be doing harm in these cases by interfering with the natural protective function of the peritoneum. In my experience, while the mortality was high in this type of patient, survivals were seen in many who were able to wall off the process. The procedure was disbanded.

A number of states now report data on surgeons' complication and mortality rates. This is particularly true for cardiac surgery. Many surgical professional organizations are tackling the problem of reporting complications to the public. It is important to remember that this often leads to the other edge of the sword, namely that surgeons may avoid operating on higher risk patients in order to lower their complication rates. While this may be a satisfactory aim for insurance companies and

Medicare, it is an attitude that may deny many patients (particularly the elderly) the benefit of appropriate treatment (see Chapter 9).

CHAPTER 5: LIFE IN ACADEMIA
THE CHAIRMAN RULES

I was hired by Clarence Dennis at SUNY Downstate for $12,000 per year, big money after my resident's pay. I arrived in the middle of June, and apparently no one knew I was coming.

There was no office, secretary or lab space. I had a lucky break, which was tragic for somebody else. The weekend before I set foot in Downstate, one of our young surgical faculty members was killed in a car accident on the Interboro Parkway. For those not from New York, this parkway consists of two narrow winding lanes through Queens separated from the oncoming traffic by a one-foot wall. The parkway was built when cars were skinny, and not meant for today's vehicles or speeds. Also, if you hit the retaining wall, there is a tendency for the wheels to run up and over, throwing the car into a lane of oncoming traffic, which is exactly what happened to our young surgeon. Killed on the spot.

I got his office, his secretary, and also his lab space.

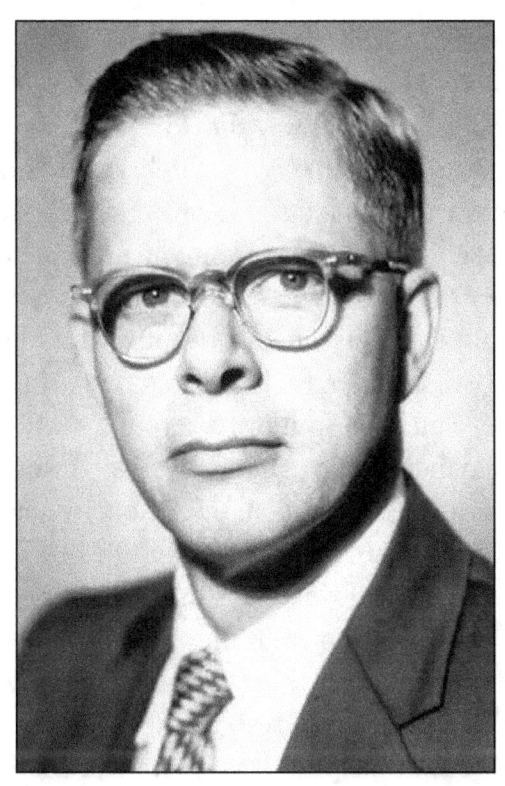

Clarence Dennis

I need to describe Downstate a bit about Downstate. The university was fairly new, although the medical school was the former Long Island College of Medicine, a stately and honored institution with a long and prominent history. It was subsequently moved from downtown Brooklyn to Flatbush, across the street from Kings County Hospital. This was once a beautiful middle-class area of Brooklyn, but when I was there, inhabited by low- income minority groups, with high unemployment and many welfare- supported families. This mirrored many of our inner cities. Typical for a state institution were the attitudes of some of the employees. My arrival in June upset their books, and the solution offered to me was to simplify their accounting by skipping my June paycheck and starting fresh in July.

The county hospital was a city-run institution, and heavily unionized. The physical plant was huge, with a 4000-bed acute care hospital, including special buildings for tuberculosis and radio-therapy—second only to Los Angeles County Hospital in size. It primarily dealt with indigent patients and was able to garner over the years a dedicated group of nurses and doctors who cared for these patients in old facilities, but providing the finest in modern care. There was a plan for a new Kings County on the city books since the middle 1930s, and still referred to when I arrived in 1965.

Repairs were held off, except for the direst circumstances, pending the building of the new hospital.

Across the street, a beautiful large medical school and a modern university hospital of only 250 beds was being completed. It was kept small in size by the political machinations of the private practitioners in Brooklyn, who feared competition from a major university on their doorstep. We never had an adequate number of beds for all of our programs. However, new lab space and offices were included in the plans.

The civil servants who staffed the non-professional core of the County Hospital were often hired to swell the union rolls, and in some instances jobs were created where none existed. The unions responded by powerful support for the mayors in their next election. While most of these workers were dedicated to their jobs and their patients, a few were not adequately trained. It was impossible to fire anyone, or to document incompetence. (Things weren't much different at the General Hospital in San Francisco, or at Bellevue, where I went to medical school.) Remember, we're talking about the 1960's and '70s.

We frequently took care of prisoners at the County. As you can guess, one of them escaped and was loose in the hospital. There was a basement that connected all of the different buildings, and that's where this fellow headed. He ran into four employees who captured the guy and had their pictures in the paper and on TV as heroes. The employees weren't supposed to be in the basement, but it was rumored that they were there playing poker when this prisoner barged in. Nobody asked embarrassing questions.

However, I must stress that we cared for a variety of major medical problems and trauma in patients that often could not afford to lose a day of work, waiting for treatment in a busy clinic. Most of the nurses, aides and social workers who worked with these patients were dedicated to their care, in spite of low remuneration.

My introduction to academic surgery was a wonderful experience, the ability to teach and scrub with the residents, teaching medical students and doing research was an entry to a world that provided a host of pleasurable stimuli. I took no vacations for the first few years, and spent many hours writing grants and papers. The atmosphere at Downstate was intoxicating; we studied all aspects of clinical surgery, made movies for meetings, and I presented talks wherever I could. But there are underlying deadly traps in academia in those days, which one may avoid by following some simple rules:

(1) Don't do a good job at committee meetings. They accomplish nothing and kill important time,

which is always in short supply. After a while, you won't be asked to serve.

(2) Don't waste time teaching medical students. Nobody cares if you are the best or worst teacher in the world. Nothing counts for academic success except publications (size of bibliography is usually more important than quality). Good teachers don't get promoted on the basis of their teaching skills.

(3) Avoid scrubbing with the residents—if you're good, they won't leave you alone.

I, and many of my surgical colleagues, never followed these precepts This meant long hours at work, including weekends. Most academic surgeons spend eighty hours a week on these endeavors. This is quite different from other specialties. I found many surgeons in other universities to be dedicated to patients and teaching.

The faculty spent an enormous amount of time and energy trying to settle our economic woes. For the 17 years I was at Downstate, we fought over this issue. It was a problem (and still is) at some medical schools. Many department chiefs have been fired over the economics of private practice. The issue is as follows:

There are three main sources of funding for medical schools. Hard money consists of a fixed budget from endowments, the government (Downstate was a state-supported school), church or philanthropic groups. Hard money is consistently stable. Soft money comes from grants-in-aid, research grants, etc., which carry salary lines for faculty, research assistants, secretarial and other personnel, as well as indirect costs which go to support labs, and the daily running costs of building maintenance, etc. Soft money depends on the efforts of faculty and administration in obtaining support for the programs and research in the school. It is, however, inconsistently available, since grants expire and need to be renewed.

When I first started out, soft money was plentiful, and large segments of faculty at many medical schools were supported by grants. As research grant money began to dry up in the late 1960s and '70s, faculty support dwindled, and other sources of funding were sought.

The third source of funding is from the private practice of the faculty. As a general rule, surgery departments are the big earners in most medical schools, although the recent ascendency of invasive specialties in cardiology, gastroenterology and radiotherapy compete for this honor.

Many faculty members in medicine and pediatrics are poor earners, either because they are reimbursed at a low rate, or they simply don't want to be bothered with patient responsibility. Deans, however, need to support these faculty members as they carry out teaching and research. The obvious answer is to harness all the practice earnings and redistribute them, a very touchy subject.

Those internists that enjoy treating private patients, and all of the surgeons, object. Surgeons will take call and handle critical patients night or day. Some trauma surgeons sleep at the hospital when on call to be better available for emergencies. They resent having to do this and have their earnings shared with faculty who are seen consistently exiting the institution at 5 o'clock. I once had a patient whom I diagnosed as acute hyperthyroidism (previously undiagnosed) and couldn't arrange for a faculty endocrinologist to see her. With cajoling and practically begging, one finally agreed, although he stated his primary interest was in patients with defects in copper metabolism (exceedingly rare).

On weekends, the hospital parking lot was loaded with the cars of surgeons, who were making rounds on their patients. Few cars of the internists, or other clinical faculty were to be seen.

An example of this was a patient of mine who had undergone an extensive cancer resection. During the first post-operative days she dropped her urinary output, and her chemistries suggested that she was going into renal failure. It was a Friday afternoon when we had the renal fellow see her for dialysis.

He agreed and said he would schedule her for Monday morning. I knew that there were significant differences in results of dialysis between chronic renal failure patients and post-operative patients. The latter group require immediate dialysis once renal failure is diagnosed, to avoid infections and other complications. I insisted that the dialysis be carried out no later than Saturday morning. It was. The patient fully recovered.

On Monday I got a phone call from the director of the dialysis unit. "You S.O.B., you're really tough," he said.

I answered, "If you needed an operation who would you want to do it?"

"You," he said.

We had another problem at Downstate. The state of New York wanted the money earned by the faculty to add to its general budget. It was felt that as state employees, we weren't entitled to our practice earnings. It didn't matter that our earnings involved many extra hours of work. This left everything in limbo for years while the problem was litigated. No one ever figured out what the claim of the state was on the efforts of the faculty in seeing private patients; after all, lawyers don't pay the state for use of the courts.

After long court wrangling and a number of newspaper articles labeling the faculty as thieves (taking state money for their own use), the state prevailed. The institution was destroyed as a referral center for many years, as the prime clinical faculty quit and moved to other institutions.

A similar battle in New Jersey was won by the faculty, which remained intact and contributed a hefty amount to the dean's fund.

This same problem played out at scores of medical schools throughout the U.S., resulting in the shifting of many chiefs of surgery from job to job. I remember getting a call from a prestigious Cleveland university to come and be their new chief of surgery—and to fire all the surgeons on the faculty. Needless to say, I wasn't interested in that job.

Some medical schools were so abusive that surgery never flourished, and recruitment of faculty was impossible. Others went through the courts, with chairmen suing deans and vice versa. Bitterness prevailed at other places. Some deans were resourceful enough to negotiate arrangements with the leading surgical earners that bypassed the practice plans, so that these specialists could be retained. This was suspected at institutions within the state system in New York. You couldn't get a straight answer on what anybody earned. There were figures quoted for publication, and the real deals.

Gradually those schools that were most successful developed practice plans that were not confiscatory to the practitioners, and an amiable compromise was reached. In many, the departments maintained their own practice funds, with a percentage payment to the dean, often redistributed to support non-earning faculty in other departments. In some, caps on earnings were installed, but in most a percentage of earnings went to administration, so that it was an advantage to have big earning departments. The most successful did away with earning caps. Retaining the clinicians' interest in teaching was sometimes accomplished by a graduated tax, increasing with increasing earnings.

The situation had gotten worse with the introduction of managed care and reduced reimbursement from government programs. Patients that were formerly going to large centers are now going elsewhere, because care is often rendered at reduced, negotiated rates, and workups may be limited by the managed care plans. New groundbreaking diagnostic techniques and treatments, often available at medical schools and large teaching hospitals, may not be reimbursed by some management or insurance plans. Hospital occupancy has decreased markedly, putting a strain on all faculty to practice in order to support the schools. Faculty who used to avoid practice by dint of their research efforts (did they hide in their laboratories?) now had to see patients if departments of medicine and pediatrics are to survive. Some of these changes are, in my opinion, good for the schools.

Another strain is government insurance in the form of Medicare and Medicaid. Reimbursement to hospitals is often reasonable, but payment for physician services is low for Medicare and practically non-existent for Medicaid. Hospitals collect a fee for Medicaid patients, and this may include physician services, precluding separate physician billing. The doctors may or may not get paid for their services from the hospitals. Worse is the creation of a large group of working poor who are not covered by either program. They earn enough in wages to be ineligible for Medicaid. They can't afford private insurance, and their only source of care is the large (usually university) hospital emergency room. When care is rendered, who foots the bill?

Sometimes the state government will pay something, usually inadequate, to cover the actual costs, leaving large deficits for the hospital. There is usually no reimbursement for the physicians. Often, the hospitals will of necessity pass this on to insurance companies which, of course, will get the money from your premiums. In other cases, patients are billed directly. The amounts can be tremendous, leaving patients thousands of dollars in debt.

Emergency rooms in many states are mandated to treat the patients that show up. In some private hospitals the patient is turned away and sent to an emergency room elsewhere, where they cannot be refused treatment.

Additionally, the training of fellows in special programs and procedures has developed a cadre of experts who practice in large teaching community hospitals, where there are no demands on their earnings. The university hospital no longer has a monopoly on some of these special programs. (Many of these community hospitals have dubbed themselves "university hospitals." This has put these hospitals in direct competition for patients with the medical schools, and they are generally better equipped to advertise and promote themselves. This necessitates rotating residents and students to busy hospitals for teaching, as the patient population in the university hospital drops.

I will get back to this in a later section.

I must add that I chaired a committee to solve the financial problem before the litigation started. We met weekly for a year and interviewed all key members of the faculty. Some of the attitudes were amazing. One famous chairman of physiology said that the clinicians should not make more money than the basic science (non-practicing) faculty, despite the extra hours of effort. When asked how these bright faculty could afford to put their children through an Ivy League college, he responded that they shouldn't aspire to such luxury if they couldn't afford it. This harkened back to the days when teaching at a medical school was a hobby for the very wealthy.

The committee came up with a solution that everyone bought into, even the basic science members. It was simply a graduated tax which limited open-ended income based on gross earnings. No allowances were made for practice expenses, but a fixed "lulu" was to be given, and practitioners could arrange their expenses any way they wished. College tuition for children of all the faculty was included. The president of the medical complex was a leader without leadership ability and hesitated long enough so that the plan died. We then went to court for ten years.

The years spent in academic surgery were glorious. Intellectually stimulating, working with like-minded colleagues developing new procedures, doing basic research and growing clinically led to a busy and productive life. I presented papers at prestigious meetings, was invited to be visiting professor at major institutions. I once had three papers accepted at the American College of Surgeons forum on fundamental research and had to race from hotel to hotel in order to present each one. The meeting was so large that even in Chicago, multiple hotels were used for the many presentations. In those days, even one paper on the forum was considered a major academic accomplishment.

In 1972 I petitioned my chairman to let me develop a surgical oncology service. This was a new concept in those days, except for the categorical cancer hospitals. He agreed over the objections of some members of the faculty, if I could demonstrate an increase in case load from the 400 cases we were currently doing annually. I started a fellowship and a computerized tumor registry, one of the first outside of a cancer hospital.

We got the hospital to let us build a small outpatient OR and hire a secretary for the service. We had a tumor registry of five secretaries on the lowest pay scale who turned over every year—impossible. I got the administration to agree to hire one secretary director and two secretaries at a higher pay scale to replace the five we had there, and they did twice the work. Those wonderful and loyal people stayed with me for the next eleven years.

Over the next few years, we did 1,200 minor surgeries a year, with the fellows training residents to do the procedures, and we did 600 major procedures in the inpatient OR.

I recruited a head and neck surgeon from the University of Texas MD Anderson Cancer Center to work on the service and when he left, another from

Memorial. This latter surgeon and I worked together for many years, and he became spectacularly successful, running his own surgical department when I left Downstate. Many years later he subsequently became chief of surgery at Downstate.

A third surgeon joined us in an interesting way. We had a large trauma service at Kings County, which admitted about two thousand cases a year. It was run by two surgeons who I will refer to as Joe and Al. These fellows had a trauma conference at which they reviewed the management of various cases and attacked each other unmercifully, a great teaching technique. It was a show at which the residents cringed but was highly attended. Immediately after the conference, we three would meet for lunch as though nothing had happened. This is a testimony to the New York attitude that criticism did not entail dislike. These fellows remained best friends throughout their careers and to this day.

I have to say something about lunch. Kings County hospital had a private dining room for faculty for many years, attended by waitresses, with table cloths, the whole schmeer, and where you could have a three-course meal for thirty cents. The food was delicious, as it had been years before at Bellevue. This luxury was subsequently phased out. Remember that we all did our stints at County without reimbursement. I never received a penny for the 1,800 cases we did yearly on our tumor service until just before I left, when I received $20,000 a year (about $11 per case).

I noticed over a period of time that Joe wasn't eating well. He began to lose weight and saw many of our specialists and nothing turned up. After some time I talked to him seriously, and found that he had scrubbed on a case with a resident, an abdominal perineal resection (to remove a rectal cancer) and felt that he was losing his talent for general surgery because of his long stint on trauma.

We arranged for him to become part of our tumor service. I put him in charge of colorectal cancer. Within a short time he regained his confidence, and subsequently became a whiz in this area, publishing a number of articles and book chapters. Unfortunately, he regained all of his lost weight and molted out of his svelte appearance.

Across the street from County was the university hospital and the medical school. The hospital had 250 beds, as I previously mentioned, due to the fear of practicing Brooklyn physicians. My introduction to practice in Brooklyn was at a dinner for the medical society. I sat next to a family practitioner, and we discussed my areas of expertise. He asked if I wanted referrals, and when I indicated my interest he asked, "What's in it for me?" I subsequently operated on two members of his family, but never saw a private referral. In fact, I operated on many physicians' family members, but never their private patients.

One of our young faculty members got the message and worked out a unique scheme. He had season tickets at the opera, pro football and a table at one of the famous restaurants in the city. Many of his referrers used these "benefits." He soon had a whopping practice.

The Markle Scholarship

I need to spend some time in describing a unique experience which was opened to a few academicians. The John and Mary Markle foundation established a fund to promote the public good, and after several undistinguished years hired John Russell as director. John believed that this small foundation could make a special impact if it developed a program to support people during their developmental stages, when they needed help, and who were likely to become leaders. He chose the medical field to do this. An elaborate plan was devised for each medical school to nominate one faculty member at the assistant professor level or below (nobody who was already established) yearly. The choice was to be someone who was likely to become a leader in academia.

These men and women met at a resort for three days in one of three sections; east, central, and west.

Some of the country's top leaders of industry, letters, arts, and politics and their spouses were selected to evaluate the candidates in each section. They were to dine, talk, engage in seminars with the candidates for the entire period with NO discussion of medical topics. It was assumed that all the candidates were competent in the medical field.

The purpose was that, after three days, these leaders would select five of the twenty or so candidates in each section to become Markle scholars, and those selected would receive $20,000 yearly as free money to use in research, or as a salary supplement to keep them in academic positions. The award was for five years.

I was selected to go as a candidate in 1968. We met in Williamsburg, Virginia and all twenty of us were petrified. We read obscure books as a preparation in order to impress our hosts with our worldliness.

The candidates' spouses were originally invited but dropped in my year because John felt that our spousal choices were all so similar that it wouldn't differentiate us. I studied Chinese history and European furniture, but the subjects never came up. It was not unusual in the middle of dinner for one of the candidates to pipe up with information about some 2,000-year-old fish which was now extinct, a topic unrelated to anything being discussed at the time.

My roommate, a surgeon from Harvard, was so nervous that he took three showers a day. I actually felt pretty relaxed.

Three months later, I was notified that I was a winner and the award would start immediately. The importance of these awards can't be overstated. Although I had a small grant at the time, this new money enabled me to expand my research and was used to pay for trips to Europe to meet other investigators, which would have been impossible otherwise.

Faculty salaries were very low, and one could make triple or quadruple the amount by going into private practice. Many good faculty were lost this way, because the demands of private practice left little time for teaching or research. In speaking to many of the other scholars, they felt that the award helped most of them through difficult times until they became established investigators and could compete for their own grants.

Membership also involved the annual scholar and spouse meeting. These were held in plush resorts (John said he wanted the scholars to see how the surgeons lived), all paid for. The meeting consisted of three days of seminars on topics chosen by the scholars (no medicine, of course), centered around the leading thinkers of the day, many of whom were invited to present at the meeting. We all received a bibliography of the works of the guests ahead of time, so we were prepared to discuss the topics. The evenings were reserved for the scholars to meet and renew friendships, many of which lasted a lifetime. These meetings were a wonderful break from the routine of academic life and kept us in touch with our developing academic world.

In the following years many of the deans, department chairmen, university presidents and leading researchers came from the ranks of the Markle scholars. Even cabinet secretaries and the director of the NIH had been scholars. When John Russell retired, a new director was hired who felt that the aim of the foundation should change. The fellowship was discontinued, and the money was used to support the media, especially public television. Many of us felt an acute loss, although federal grant support had increased at that time. Now, with the later drastic cutbacks in research support, and with the push to practice, many faculty are finding it difficult to remain in academics. A smaller version of the Markle program was started by Johnson & Johnson, but with less impact.

As noted earlier, we did a large and varied number of operations on our service, and we made several movies of procedures that were presented at national and international meetings. I had my children work in the lab one summer, memories that lasted many years for them. I was blessed with a dedicated lab technician who was a whiz with small animals. We did most of our research with rats, rabbits and prairie dogs. I hired a Ph.D. chemist, who worked with me for many years and subsequently went on to become professor of chemistry at a New York college. He was an African-American who had a serious limp from polio as a child. He had been hospitalized for over a year as a teenager, and his mother continued his education by bringing him books and studying with him daily. She was not well-educated but made the effort. He stands as a monument to what the human heart and mind can accomplish. He subsequently moved to a teaching position at a university.

When he left, my luck held out and I hired an Egyptian chemistry Ph.D. who was brilliant in analyzing the metabolism of cholesterol in the liver and its effect on bile metabolism. He found another academic position in the City University of New York when I left Downstate, and had been promoted to associate professor there. His twin daughters became physicians.

I received a letter from a Swiss surgeon, Rollf Muller, who applied for a fellowship to join our tumor service. He had been working in Africa with Albert Schweitzer, operating on African patients who needed his skills. I hired him, and several months later he was joined by his girlfriend, a lovely Swiss nurse. As with all my fellows, they attended dinners at our home periodically.

As the year ended, they decided to marry in New York. I found a pastor through the Ethical Culture Society, and with us as witnesses they were married in a simple but beautiful ceremony. We then went to a well- known Argentinian restaurant near Rockefeller center for our wedding meal. With difficulty, we were able to communicate with the Spanish speaking staff and had a delicious dinner. For desert they brought a lovely cake with a candle. As they placed this on the table, a group of waiters appeared and began singing "Happy Birthday." I guess our communication skills were somewhat ineffective.

I had a fellow from Japan, Jiro Fugimoto, who was an excellent surgeon. He worked with our residents, and he and his wife Taeko joined us in parties we held for students and residents on our service. He rose to fame in Osaka and I was dismayed at never making the trip to Japan. He and I communicate by snail mail each year to this day.

We traveled to Bangkok one year to give a lecture at a major hospital. A former fellow, Dr. Niminnet, was in practice north of the city, and he and his wife insisted on taking us around. This was a blessing, since the traffic in the city was unbearable. He had a relative who was a couturier and very well known. My daughter Karen, was to be married in several months, so Joan had a gown made for the wedding. With several visits for measuring, it was a knockout.

Travel to various countries was necessary to maintain one's reputation, and to see what was developing at other universities. Getting away allowed time to rejuvenate after a series of eighty-hour weeks. Whenever possible, we tied our vacation time to meetings and presentations.

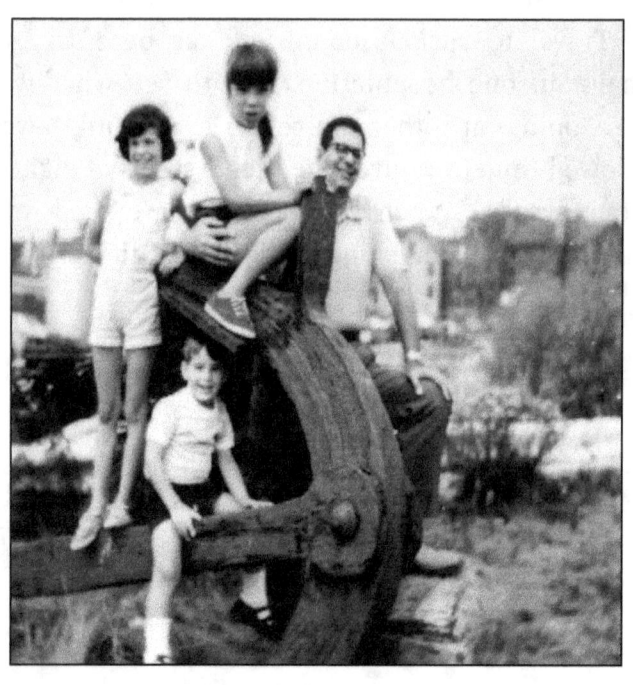

Traveling with the children was always a treat for Joan and me.

Sometimes we hired nannies to stay with our children, and as they got older we would take them along. In those days, the economies of European countries were well below the U.S., enabling cheaper hotel and travel costs, particularly Italy, France and Spain. My university salary was my main income source in spite of a large practice. Most of my patients were from lower income groups, and I stayed within their insurance parameters. Fortunately, I had excellent grant support which often included money for travel, although within tight federal limits.

I was asked to deliver a paper on my research on gall stone dissolution using heparin. This treatment necessitated the insertion of a tube into a duct feeding the gallbladder. The treatment was successful, and some years later a system of trans-duodenal insertion was developed by the gastroenterologists and radiologists, which greatly simplified the treatment of this condition.

The meeting was in Davos, Switzerland. My sister and brother-in-law came along for a drive through France, stopping in towns with a Michelin-awarded restaurant. My sister would take two to three suitcases for a weekend trip, so you can imagine what she carried to France. We planned to finish in San Remo, Italy, after which they would go home, and Joan and I would proceed to Davos.

We arrived in Paris to claim the Hertz rented car. Hertz said they never made the reservation. My brother-in-law and I went to the top of the parking garage and started walking down. We found a Ford station wagon in an upper floor and rented it.

One day, we passed through a small town and registered at a hotel. As is usual in France, the men watched and the ladies carried all the luggage to our room. The next morning, after a glorious meal the previous night, we started packing the car. We noticed that the entire staff of the hotel was lined up on the street watching us load. Now Irv and I had worked out a system so we knew where each piece of luggage would just fit. As we finished and began locking up, the entire staff burst into applause. I guess there were doubts about our ability to get everything in.

In San Remo, we visited a casino. It was our last night before splitting up. We were not allowed to sit at the tables (reserved for the townspeople), but could place bets by standing behind them. I had an unbelievable streak of luck, guessing correctly fifteen consecutive times. I left the next day carrying thousands of Italian lire as Joan and I went on to Switzerland.

We stayed with the Mullers (my former fellow) who now had a booming practice. They had a very pretty and very advanced home in Altdorf, in which everything worked with buttons, opening doors and windows electrically. There was a heated pool in the basement which could be opened by pressing another button. Altdorf was high in the Alps, and Rolff, who was a long-distance skier, spent each morning skiing and seeing patients in the afternoons. He discussed the medical system in Switzerland. Everyone had some coverage. For surgery there were three levels, (1) the trained residents operated, (2) A private surgeon in practice scrubbed to assist the resident, and (3) the private surgeon took total control of the case. No patient was devoid of coverage.

I told Rolff of my luck in San Remo and asked how I could get rid of the lire. He took me to his bank where the officer told me that I could not leave Italy with so many lire as it was against the law. When I asked what I could do, he answered "Open an account." That's how I got a Swiss bank account. It amounted to about $3,500 American. I kept it several years when I realized I was losing money on it and I transferred the money to my US bank.

The next morning we drove to Davos. Each morning the ranchers drove a long line of cattle with clanking bells around their necks up to the mountains to graze, and back to their barns in the evening.

My paper was pleasantly received and the x-rays of patients undergoing the heparin treatment were reviewed and the results confirmed.

Many practicing surgeons don't understand the demands of academic life. We had an old-time busy surgeon who was on the voluntary faculty, frequently scrubbing with the trauma residents. He was not boarded in surgery and felt that this was unfair to the residents he assisted. In order for him to qualify for the surgical boards, he had to return to a residency for a year, which he did. This is extremely difficult for a busy surgeon to do. It meant giving up his practice and working beside a resident you had recently supervised in the OR. He never complained about night call or hard work, passed his boards, and returned to practice.

However, he asked for an appointment to the full-time faculty and was happily appointed. After a year on the faculty, he resigned with the comment that he had never worked so hard in his life. Private practice was a snap for him, and he returned to his former schedule.

Incidentally he became jaundiced (turned yellow) in later years and was convinced he had a pancreatic cancer. He refused treatment and kept operating until he developed cholangitis with a high fever. I operated and found a common duct with stones and an abnormal connection between the duct and the intestinal tract (a fistula). He actually did very well after repair and returned to full time practice.

CHAPTER 6: MOVING TO A PRIVATE-PRACTICE (TEACHING) HOSPITAL

During my stay at Downstate, I had interviewed for many chairman positions around the country. One in particular was noteworthy. The chairman of the search committee met me at the airport of this midwestern city, and we had dinner at his home. He had just shot a duck that day and cooked it. I felt these small metal pellets in my mouth, which I unobtrusively spit into my napkin. I guess he really did shoot it. The guests told me about the lack of teenage crime in this town. It seems that as soon as the children are able, they leave town for more exciting places. Needless to say, when I discussed this with Joan we eliminated that job.

Many of the institutions I went to had multiple serious problems with salary levels, administrators that felt that private practice earnings should pay for the clinic cleanup crews and such, and deans who were ravenous in their attempts to garner the income of surgeons for their own benefits. As a result, some of these institutions developed weak departments made up of surgeons that didn't care to operate much, and therefore resident training was left to community hospitals through which the residents rotated. As we will see, this is a bad environment for resident training, because the stress is on referral of patients and fees and not on teaching.

Joan and I both felt an obligation to bring up our children in a stable environment, and as a result I never seriously looked at moving away from the New York area and our relatives and friends. I now advise students interested in academic careers to plan at least two or three moves to provide recognition nationally and promotions. They must be available to go wherever their careers lead them.

In 1981 I received a letter from a large private hospital looking for a chief of surgery. I made my usual one trip to the facility, met a lot of people, left and turned down the job. They continued their search without much luck.

About a year-and-a-half later, I got a call from the CEO to please come and have dinner with him and the chairman of the board at a restaurant of my choice in the city. Joan and I talked things over. We had saved some money, but hardly enough to put our kids through a decent college, much less plan for our retirement. Pam was at the University of Wisconsin, Karen was recently married at a very expensive affair, and Robbie was going to finish high school soon. And to boot, we had a new chairman who was a clod in dealing with people and jealous of our surgical oncology division. He was going to break it up to enhance his own expertise.

I got a call from Ben Rush, the chairman of surgery at the New Jersey medical school who used the hospital as a full affiliate. He guaranteed to rotate fifteen residents through the program there and to give me full support. In addition, he offered a full professorship on an academic tenured line. This would be the first tenured position outside the university campus.

When we looked at all aspects of the problem, I decided to have the dinner at the Perigord East, my favorite restaurant. I wasn't going to take the job and determined to ask for an exorbitant deal. At dinner, everything I asked for was granted, including a super retirement package, high salary, private practice income and an assortment of benefits. One disturbing fact, however, came up. I was asked if I would take the job in the face of a petition signed by the department members saying that they didn't want me. They had never met me, and I figured that they were frightened that I would arrive with a bunch of new staff that would threaten their practices. I said I could handle it if the board

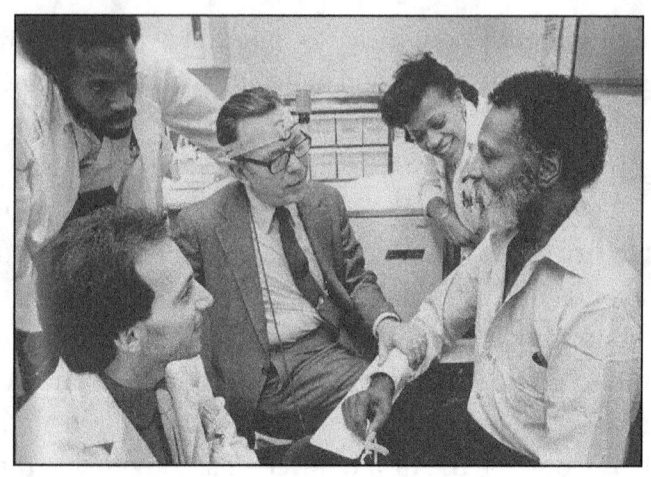

Dr. Ben Rush, the man who brought me to Jersey

would support me. This optimistic view, however, was later to be severely challenged. I took the job.

We moved in January of 1983. Joan had looked at 34 houses, starting as close to the George Washington Bridge as she could get. Gradually she moved west and found a beautiful house on a lake. We were at the height of the real estate depression, and high interest rates and two circumstances combined to make our choice possible.

One member of the board was a bank president, who provided us with a reduced-rate mortgage as an incentive to take the job. The second was that the builders had built this house on speculation and were paying enormous interest rates over the three years of its existence. They had house sitters to keep things in shape. They had to reduce the price in order to sell it. We borrowed money from my sister to bridge the period until our house in Cedarhurst was sold.

We arrived with our movers and were greeted by our real estate agent and her husband, who was by coincidence a member of the board at this hospital. To our surprise, our house sitters had removed the refrigerator, which apparently belonged to them, and I ran out and bought one that afternoon. The agent and her husband, who subsequently became our closest friends, brought Chinese food for dinner while the movers unpacked.

The acting chairman of surgery had arranged for several of my visits to meet people on the staff and administration. His secretary was inefficient and confused dates and times. In any case, I determined to hire a new secretary on whom I could count for loyalty. I interviewed a lady who had limited experience in the medical field but had worked as chief administrator for a bank president in the area. She had retired, but shortly afterwards her husband died of a heart attack. They were in their forties.

She tried traveling, being with her children, church activities but to no avail. She was depressed and lonely, and now was trying to get back in the workforce. I hired her, and she developed into the best secretary I ever had. We subsequently hired other secretaries to help run the department, which involved resident training, student teaching, administration, clinical research and my private practice. From the start, she did everything and never complained about the volume of work. Keeping my calendar alone was a major job, since I was a member and officer of many local and national societies, presenting lectures and papers at many meetings, and involved in innumerable meetings at the hospital.

I had a private practice at Downstate along with teaching, research, publishing papers, traveling to scientific meetings, etc. However, surgeons practicing as their only activity were driven by the elements of earnings and local prestige, which I soon appreciated.

In order to better understand the motivating forces within the hospital, it's important to focus on the ground rules of private practice.

Patients are the key. They represent a commodity which determines the politics and power of the staff members. The doctor with the most patients is the most powerful. At our hospital, the patient belonged to the first doctor who saw him. This rule is carried to extremes so, for example, a patient who appears at the emergency room with some problem is always asked if they have ever seen a doctor on the staff. If so, that doctor is contacted, regardless of the complaint. Suppose the patient is having abdominal pain and needs a surgeon. None is called until the family practitioner that the patient saw three years ago is called. He or she then makes the referral to a specific surgeon, and the ER nurse makes the contact. This resulted in a near-tragedy one day, when a young girl was seen with a severe head injury. Because she was operated upon by a neurosurgeon at the hospital years earlier, the call went out to him. He was not available on beeper and could not be reached, despite the fact that the neurosurgeon on call was in the hospital at the time. The patient did poorly while waiting, although she survived. We subsequently changed the rules for true emergencies.

The family practitioners or internists have the greatest power, because they control most of the referrals and most of the beds in the hospital. Surgeons in practice over a long period may develop a large patient-to-patient referral system. They become powerful because they have patients to refer to medical specialists, i.e. cardiologists or gastroenterologists. Clearly, the practitioner with the most referrals to make controls the power. Most surgeons depend on referrals, and therefore are at the mercy of the family practitioners, which incidentally may include internists and other medical specialists. Although surgeons at many hospitals may be loud and boisterous, they will toe the line when it comes to any confrontation with the hospital administration and can be counted on to support the medical staff.

A problem arises when the hospital is the first to see the patient, e.g. in a clinic or emergency room manned by salaried ER doctors, or even worse, by practitioners (any specialty) salaried by the hospital. The control of that commodity now leaves the private practice arena and becomes currency of use to the hospital. This, therefore, puts the hospital in direct competition for patients. The staff will never refer a patient to a hospital-based physician unless there is no equivalent expert on the staff.

Even under those circumstances, the referral may be made to another large teaching hospital well out of the referring area, which gives the patients the sense that their doctor really cares to get the best specialist, while guaranteeing that the patients will return to his care when they get home. This in spite of the fact that there may be as competent a specialist on the salaried physician staff.

This may not pertain if the salaried physician stays strictly within his specialized area and does not compete with a staff doctor. An example may be a transplant program where the transplant team is salaried and doesn't do anything else. If one of these surgeons should perform a hernia or gastrectomy for example, it would not be surprising to see patients referred elsewhere for transplantation.

The hospital administration, of course, would love to control its own patient load and not be beholden to the staff to fill its beds. So there is a constant battle with the private practitioners to develop programs that the administration can control. Some hospitals have worked out appropriate compromises to guarantee staff independence. But the staff is always on the lookout for subtle intrusions into what it considers its domain, the private practice of medicine. Sometimes the staff may mobilize, leave and open its own hospital (doctors' hospitals in some areas).

In some places, this is described as the "town-gown" problem, but it is ultimately derived from the economics of practice. This was why the university hospital at Downstate was limited to 250 beds, and why the practitioners sent me their relatives but not their patients. At many major university hospitals, patient referrals come from out-of-state or long distances, rather than from the local communities.

These systems change in some areas where the teaching hospital survives. The hospital may be strong enough to buy the practices of physicians and pay salaries to assure admissions. Newer ideas may use the presence of hospitalists (paid physicians) to care for inpatients, with on-call specialists or groups acting as consultants (see Chapter 9).

When I arrived, the administration and staff were entwined in a struggle to dominate the responsible board of the hospital. Most voluntary hospitals have a group of well-known local citizens who have the fiscal responsibility for the institution, which is theoretically non-profit. They may be local bank presidents, automobile dealers, etc. who make up the trustees. Sometimes they go by other names, i.e. managers or regents, etc. Since these are busy people, they elect an executive committee to oversee the problems with the hospital and its function. They, in fact, represent the ultimate decision power of the institution.

This board hires the CEO (chief administrator of the hospital), and he hires a staff of other administrators and personnel to do the daily chores such as the admissions office, record room, laundry, repairs, patient payments, etc. These administrators are highly paid and their boss, the CEO, deals directly with the trustees, giving them information when necessary at scheduled meetings. But he is not their only source of information. Many members of the board or their families get sick and are cared for by members of the medical staff. Board members may, on many occasions, meet with staff members socially and then get fed other information, which at times may be in direct conflict with that from the CEO.

The medical staff has direct control of the medical affairs of the hospital, such as privileges of its members (what they are allowed to do), and who may admit and treat patients at the hospital, and all the medical activities that go on daily. It does this through a series of committees, all of which report to an elected medical board which meets monthly or more often.

This board takes the reports of the committees and their recommendations and decides what needs to be done to facilitate the operations of the hospital, and the CEO is required to carry out the recommendations. Since the staff is diverse and busy, it usually will allow a medical board elected from its members to make all the important decisions and to look out for its interests. Department chairmen, some of whom may be salaried by the hospital, serve on this board. Thus, the exact composition of the board will determine who controls the hospital.

The interests of the staff revolve around income. It is to their interest to keep competing physicians off the staff. Many ruses are used to accomplish this. Incoming physicians must have offices in the immediate community (to avoid incoming experts from the big city getting on staff and stealing patients). A stringent set of qualifications and credentials are required to prolong the process. Excuses are often found why a particular physician cannot get on staff.

For years at my new hospital, department chairmen (professors at the medical school), who often sent residents for training, could only come on the staff as consultants when asked (no admitting privileges to avoid competition with the staff). A major activity involved the local lawyers, who made a fortune out of suing the hospital to obtain staff privileges for their clients. Most applicants just gave up. Those who sued usually won, but it became generally conceded that membership on the staff might require an expensive legal foray. These same mechanisms may act politically to limit admission for practice, i.e. to physicians who perform abortions, as seen in many states.

But the medical board also protected the staff's interests against the hospital. For example, bringing in new doctors to run the clinics, or paid physicians to set up new programs, was strongly resisted. If these people could not pass the scrutiny of the medical board, they were rejected. Even programs so mundane as improving the appearance of the emergency room were turned down, for fear that a new emergency room would attract patients away from the local practitioners.

Therefore, a major controversy concerned the number of medical board members that would come from the ranks of paid physicians (department chairs, and special program leaders hired by the hospital), as opposed to the number coming from the medical staff. Clearly, a majority voting on issues as a block would give control of the hospital to the CEO (who, after all, paid the salaries of the chairmen) or to the staff.

The trustees, who had the final say washed their hands of the problem and let the battle play out in the hallways of the hospital. I, coming in as a new department chair, sided naively with the administration. I honestly felt that the hospital was entering a new era, and that I could best serve the interests of my department by this means. There wasn't much support for that view, and the rancor that developed because of the failure of the trustees failed to take definitive action lingered for a long time. The staff retained control of the institution.

When the CEO wanted to hire a group to run the emergency room, a long series of hearings and meetings ensued to guarantee that these new doctors would not see patients that "belonged" to a staff member without his (her) permission. They were also limited in what they could do with patients. For example, they were not permitted to insert chest tubes for emergent thoracic conditions, even though they were specially trained to do this, and in fact were boarded in emergency medicine. Some staff members who used to take emergency calls sued, because their jobs were taken away. They weren't trained in emergency care and some were mediocre doctors, in my opinion. They lost the suit.

I got into trouble early by trying to improve patient care in three areas.

In those days, special trauma programs were developed because of the recognized need for experts in this field to save the lives of trauma victims. Many states had conceived of the need for trauma centers and legislated levels to which patients could be directed when severely injured. In New Jersey, these designations were already being discussed, and a helicopter transport service was being developed. I decided to bring a trauma specialist on staff and to give him minimal support to upgrade our care of these patients. Our surgeons were taking trauma calls, and often some were inadequately trained to care for the major injuries we were seeing. This again led to a series of hearings which finally ended up with my adding the trauma surgeon and a special trauma nurse with a guarantee that it would not interfere with the call schedule. This man did an outstanding job of updating our trauma care and educating our surgeons. It cost me months of grief and abuse by the staff for bringing him on board.

It might be worthwhile to define the methods of abuse. First, at a weekly department meeting, I was asked to defend my decision to bring on a new staff member. Remember that the staff committees could reject the credentials of the candidate, tying him up in expensive litigation for months or years.

Second, the word got out to the rest of the staff that I was not playing by the rules, and this cut off referrals.

Third, I would have visiting professors over for dinner at my home prior to their giving grand rounds at the hospital. If I invited members of my staff, some would agree to come and then not show up, leaving my wife and me embarrassed at a dinner party. I subsequently invited only members of the faculty at the medical school who I knew would be happy to come and meet these prominent surgeons. In addition, at a staff meeting they would make up lies about my treatment of patients and accuse me of hiding my complications. The abusive language at these meetings got very personal, so even my secretary would lower her head in shame.

A second problem at the hospital was the surgical ICU (intensive care unit). Our surgeons were doing major surgery and the ICU was just a place where the nurses took more blood pressures than they did on the floor units.

The nurses were disheartened because they were aware of new techniques and principles of monitoring and treating critically ill patients that were not being used at this hospital. The surgeons would call medical specialists to care for the lungs, another to care for the heart, possibly a third to check on the antibiotics, etc., and providing consultations for a host of future referrers, while the patient was getting disjointed care. New techniques of continuous oxygen monitoring, evaluating cardiac function, ventilator support and computer programs were irregularly being used. I determined to bring in a surgical critical care specialist on a paid, full-time basis.

I found a candidate trained at Mount Sinai in New York who was willing to come. After months of arguments and petitions by my staff (a favorite mechanism), we negotiated a compromise. Our candidate could come and be in charge of the ICU, train the nurses, but not decide who could be admitted to the unit. In addition, she could not take clinic assignments or see consultations by any staff member outside the unit. There was a great fear that if she should develop a private practice, she might be a preferred referral because of her expertise in caring for critical patients. Furthermore, she could only care for patients in the unit if the surgeon gave her permission.

Despite of all the restrictions, she came and brought the whole unit into the current century. Some surgeons (the busiest) continued to practice in the old-fashioned way but allowed the nurses to utilize some of the improved methods our new director had introduced. She left the hospital when I did, after undergoing continued criticism of her methods and techniques by our surgeons, who sometimes had really limited expertise. Most of these surgeons depended on the rotating residents to take care of their patients using the new techniques developed at the medical school. Those residents loved working with our director and learned a lot from her.

At one of our famous staff meetings she was subjected to abusive language accusing her of trying to manage patients on her own. It took our cardiac surgeon to quell the rhetoric and support her monitoring methods.

A third area of concern was the burn service. Traditionally in many institutions, burns were managed by plastic surgeons. At our hospital there was a roster already established which included several of our general surgeons and all of the plastic surgeons. Burn patients require an enormous amount of expertise in management, as the mortality is established early with the initial treatment. Unless this is done correctly, the severely burned patient is not likely to survive. That's why burn patients are referred to specialized centers where expertise is available. There is a special Burn Society in surgery for those with particular interest in this area.

Burns are also a lucrative area of income for surgeons, since they require multiple operations and skin grafting as well as reconstructions. These may extend over years. Our plastic surgeons refused to give up the burn call in spite of problems in the early phases of treatment. Some residents complained about the shoddy treatment many of these patients received. Some of these surgeons refused to come in and see the patients during the acute phase. This was inexcusable. It was up to me to get them off call.

I started by accumulating the data on their treatment. With great trepidation I faced them and got the worst performers to resign from the service. This took a great deal of cajoling and threats of exposure. My usual ploy was that I would present their complications in conference, and that I would ask a medical board committee to review their work. Although they would probably be exonerated the first time or two, after a while some real questions would come up. They couldn't resist losing their regular referrals over this issue, and several of these fellows resigned, leaving a better call schedule and a safer one for the patients. The plastic surgeons never forgave me, and subsequently lined up with my surgical enemies to petition me out of the chairmanship.

I should mention at this time something about the support of the legal profession in Bergen County. Everyone on staff had his own lawyer and sued at the drop of a hat if things didn't go right. For example, if I named someone as chief of a division, two other members of that division were sure to sue. If someone wanted to bring on a partner and the other members of the section or department opposed it (Why invite competition?), there was sure to be a lawyer and a threatened suit. If one of our surgeons lost his temper in the ER and cussed out a nurse, I would have him into my office to admonish him about such behavior in front of patients. The next day, I was sure to get a letter from his lawyer. When I finally left I had several outstanding suits against me and other full-time staff members. None were ever prosecuted.

I brought on certain other surgeons to fill areas where I thought we had a weakness and to revitalize the staff. Each one was a major fight and an embarrassing department meeting. And each one added another enemy to my list.

For example, we had a pediatric surgeon who did everything including pediatric surgery. He was often unavailable, or on vacations, and would ask another surgeon to cover him who unfortunately had no training in pediatric surgery. On one occasion, a newborn infant was scheduled for surgery by our covering surgeon. I was informed by the pediatrician of the impending disaster and cancelled the case. We had the patient transferred to another facility with an available pediatric surgeon who correctly managed the problem.

The pediatricians were upset about the lack of coverage. As I usually did in these cases, I met with our surgeon and asked him to take a partner to protect his practice. There was plenty of work to go around. We had brought in a pediatric oncology group who were getting loads of referrals, and they were livid about our surgical coverage. Our surgeon refused to do this. His argument was that if he brought on a partner specifically trained in pediatric surgery, he might lose his pediatric referral sources because of his other surgical interests, and that the new man would get to be known as the real pediatric surgeon. I brought on a pediatric surgeon independently – another enemy.

A Grand Scheme

I want to describe a series of incidents now, which will portray the tenor of private practice at this hospital.

There was a family practitioner on the staff who had a fairly large practice at this and another hospital, where several of our surgeons also practiced.

I was having lunch with several staff members when I noticed an unusual amount of discussion going on in the lunchroom. It seemed that a new group had been formed under the auspices and direction of this practitioner, which purported to be a multi-specialty HMO. Many of the specialists, including several of our surgeons, were on the list. The practitioner opened an outpatient center on a large highway near the hospital and offered multiple specialty services. On the surface, this was all okay. My suspicions were aroused when our neurosurgeon flew back from Florida and insisted that his name be deleted from the list, claiming that it was included without his knowledge or permission.

My second in command, who remained a friend, inquired into the arrangements for this group and came to me to tell me that he thought it was very suspicious. Apparently, the head of the group set up a billing and collection service so that every patient referred to a specialist had to be billed by this service, which would retain up to 40% of the collection as its fee. It was not clear to me whether these referrals were to be limited to patients seen at the outpatient center, or others from his other offices. It seemed to me that 40% as a billing fee was exorbitant when all these specialists had their own offices and billing staffs.

I called a meeting of the department to indicate that although I had no inclination of any impropriety, that if there was to be a problem it would reflect on the whole department. The members then voted that all outside arrangements with HMOs for each member was to be kept on file in the surgery department. My assistant director wrote a letter to the American College of Surgeons asking for their opinion on the arrangement. They responded that they did not get involved with ethical opinions but indicated that 40% seemed high for a billing service.

I got to meet the practitioner for the first time. He barged into my office with his lawyer and indicated that I was interfering with his business, and if I persisted there would be dire consequences. Since there were rumors that some of the front money for the enterprise may have been from outside sources, I wasn't certain what the form of the action would be. This meeting was followed by a warning letter from his lawyer, threatening a suit.

I then wrote a letter to the attorney for the state medical society, describing in theoretical terms the arrangement and asking his opinion. In no uncertain terms he said that the arrangement smacked of fee-splitting, and he would not recommend that doctors get involved.

I called several members of the department who were participants and showed them the letter from the attorney. They resigned from the group. In no way did I ever try to personally influence them. I didn't have the power to influence their decisions. In asking about the arrangements, the 40% figure was confirmed, although no member would give me a copy of the contract. They all knew that Medicare patients were involved and that there were strict constraints on money to referring physicians under the Medicare regulations.

I found out that the physician had made an arrangement with a cardiac group in Newark, bypassing our cardiac surgeon, who was world-renowned and who refused to participate. One member of that group was on our staff as a thoracic surgeon but did not have cardiac privileges. I spoke to him, showing him the letters, and he admitted that although they were not using the physician's HMO they agreed on a billing fee (less than 40%). With fees for cardiac surgery running into many thousands of dollars, this was a coup.

The hospital board and their attorney were getting very antsy about this time and were concerned how they would appear if word got out about the arrangements.

Then a catastrophe occurred. One of the physician's partners admitted a man with hypotension and a large thoracic aneurysm. The diagnosis was delayed a day because of a questionable x-ray reading. Informally, one of our thoracic surgeons reviewed the films and correctly told the family practitioner to call our cardiac surgeon immediately. The patient was in severe distress. Instead of calling our cardiac surgeon, they decided to transfer the patient to Newark by ambulance (a half-hour to 40-minute trip) and called their surgeons to accept the patient. The patient subsequently died at the Newark hospital.

This was inexcusable. When the word got out, a full-scale investigation of the entire HMO scheme was undertaken by the board of trustees. All hearings were held in absolute privacy, and no leaks occurred. I was not privy to any of the discussions. This went on for weeks and led to mass resignations from the HMO by involved staff members, which included partners of our chief of medicine.

The incident of the patient transfer was investigated separately by the medical department and no direct fault was found, only poor judgment.

When the hospital's board completed their investigation, a copy of the conclusions was sent to the state board of medical examiners. The staff resented the activities of the hospital trustees, judging it to be interference with the practice of medicine. The state board conducted its own inquiry, which was weak and ineffectual. One of their investigators had to be replaced, and there was a rumor of coercion or interference by the physician under investigation. Their conclusion resulted in an admonishment to him, and a description of what requirements were necessary in establishing an HMO. They carefully indicated that fees for referring patients were not included.

Then the physician sued.

Named as defendants in the suit were the president of the board, chief hospital administrator, department chairmen, the head of cardiology and probably several other staff members I can't recall. The claim was that we interfered with his business enterprise and the economic development of his HMO.

The suit was originated in state court, and the board recognized that in New Jersey this might be a risky business. There was little oversight, and we feared that the physician was well-enough connected to get a favorable judge. Our first move was to have the suit removed to federal court. This was easily done, since many of the issues involved fundamental Constitutional rights.

Then began a year-long round of depositions, which for the most part were attempts to intimidate the defendants in the hopes that the hospital would settle. My deposition was particularly grueling, since the physician was convinced that I instigated the whole mess. I was characteristically blunt in my answers, and when asked if I thought that the scheme was akin to fee splitting I answered "Absolutely!" In my mind, a 30-or 40-percent billing fee for referring patients despite of the fact that every one of the specialists had his own billing service, the differing arrangements with members of the group, the fact that in many cases no fees were even returned to the specialists, and the transfer of the critically ill patient to a member of the group all added up to a refined case of fee splitting, in my opinion.

Every once in a while, the physician would turn to his lawyer and say

"Now we've got him."

Our lawyers entered a plea for summary judgment to a spectacular and well-known judge who investigated every aspect of the case. The plaintiffs had engaged an economic expert to frame an argument concerning the loss of money and the impact of such a plan on the economy. He also accused me and the chief of cardiology of engaging in a scheme to defraud patients undergoing cardiac surgery.

The judge issued a summary judgment in our favor, except for one or two minor points which were not in his jurisdiction and were remanded to state court at the discretion of the plaintiff. His analysis of the details of the scheme was biting and hard-hitting, agreeing with all of our points. He referred to the economic analysis as juvenile. He chastised several of the doctors who testified for the plaintiff (they still were looking for referrals) as giving testimony that changed from time to time (bordering on perjury). He cleared me and the chief of cardiology of any wrongdoing.

It was a devastating defeat for this practitioner, and he never carried forth any action in state court, although he tried in many ways to continue a vendetta against me and the cardiologist.

Here is a quote from the judge's decision, which covered 127 typewritten pages:

Conclusion
"To summarize, plaintiffs' Section 1 claim for conspiracy to restrain trade is dismissed both because they cannot demonstrate the existence of an antitrust conspiracy among the defendants as a matter of law, and because their failure to present a viable market analysis prevents them from demonstrating

the existence of anti-competitive effects. Plaintiffs' Section 2 claim for a conspiracy to monopolize is also dismissed because plaintiffs' cannot prove the existence of a conspiracy... All antitrust claims must be dismissed... all state antitrust claims should be dismissed as well...

With regard to the cardiac surgery conspiracy:

"According to the records and documents submitted by both plaintiffs and defendants, HCSS is a non-profit New Jersey corporation created to receive and administer funds for scientific, educational and charitable purposes... No individual receives any of these funds. The HCSS was investigated by the medical board and found to be ethical and lega... Thus the plaintiffs' claim that the pump supervision is a source of private economic gain for Dr._____(chief of cardiology) or Dr._____(chief of surgery) is utterly baseless."

The decision resulted in a sigh of relief for the hospital and staff, an ending to a bad experience that no one wanted to relive.

We suffered some more embarrassment concerning the cardiac support services issue. An anonymous tip (guess who) to the FBI precipitated an investigation by HCFA that resulted in a demand to return Medicare fees paid for this service. The decision was based on the claim that we used incorrect codes in billing for the service. In fact, we had gotten the correct codes in writing from the insurance carriers representing Medicare. The government lawyers said that the carriers made a mistake and we had to return the money. Our lawyers indicated that the government had the right to do this under a theory called recoupment.

The hospital was in no way going to fight another legal battle, particularly when the government lawyers started to leak information to the press. We settled and disbanded the services. We repaid about $500,000 from the funds we were saving to develop a research program at the hospital.

Then an anonymous source reported the settlement to Channel 7 news, who broadcast an exposé without ever talking to any of the principals. No one familiar with the details was interviewed. They, of course, never got the details right. That series of exposés was soon discontinued.

However, a tape of the broadcast was anonymously sent to the medical school dean and to my department chairman when I returned to the medical school. I think it was also sent to the state board of medical examiners. My chairman confronted me with this information, but no one else had the courage to do this. He accepted my explanation of the service and that of the chairman of the board at the private hospital, who told everyone of the misinterpretation by HCFA, and that all of these activities were found to be ethical and legal previously by several lawyers. Especially noteworthy was the fact that no monies were ever spent for individual reimbursement. The only amount ever used was for the support of an anesthesia fellowship.

The reporter from Channel 7 never did a follow-up report on TV, and to this day I am sorry that I never sued to clear up the inferences.

This was a tough lesson for me. After seeing the activity of prosecuting lawyers personally, who refused to consider exculpatory facts, and being told by our lawyers, with extensive government experience, not to confront them since they could develop a mental set for conviction, I looked upon government announcements with suspicion. Especially when many people who fought them ruined their careers and lives, even though found innocent.

It was clear to me by this time that I was losing touch with academic surgery. I had been moving up the ranks in the Society of Surgical Oncology and was scheduled to become president. I was also on a select committee of the American College of Surgeons dealing with HCFA and reimbursement issues. I was also scheduled to become a governor of the college.

In dealing with the surgeons in the department at that hospital, there were a number of things that stood out. Their main interest was in getting referrals, and many times this was at the expense of self-education. A few may have not been up-to-date on new developments and were refractory to any criticism for fear that others in the department would talk of their problems in the halls of the hospital. They were, of course, right.

As a result, we could not run a mortality and morbidity conference by considering the errors in practice that were committed. This conference is the only one mandated to be conducted as part of all surgical training programs. It is a prime teaching vehicle to point out management problems that could be avoided in future cases. (I discussed this in a section of a previous chapter.)

In addition, some of the department members refused to go to national meetings for fear that they would lose referrals if they left town. This is not so in many other departments, because of partnerships which foster cross-coverage. Even within the few existing partnerships, there was extensive competition for cases. The American Board of Surgery recognized these problems and developed a program of reexaminations for all surgeons every ten years from their initial passing of the boards.

I tried to remedy the situation by bringing in bright young people to help fertilize the staff with new ideas. This was perceived as a threat to their practices. It was clear that if I was going to maintain any credibility, the time had come for me to return to the academic fold by joining the faculty full-time at the university.

To undermine my support from the board, the staff attacked my integrity and teaching ability unmercifully and drew up another petition, this time signed by a small majority of the members of the department. They were petrified at the thought that I would have gained a majority support. Closed hearings were held and accusations were made which I was given no chance to refute. I wasn't even present when these were aired. Upon resigning, I obtained a letter from the CEO indicating my value to the hospital and my outstanding teaching credentials and a good severance agreement. This is not an unusual event in large teaching hospitals.

During this time, a good friend of mine became chief of surgery at another major New Jersey hospital. We decided to have a meeting of chairmen in similar positions to discuss mutual problems. We invited seven other chairmen of programs in large teaching hospitals in New York, Pennsylvania, and Delaware. We met in New York City at the office of another friend who was recently appointed to a similar position. After an afternoon of extended talk and sharing of views, we met our wives and had a catered dinner at Le Cirque in Manhattan.

All of us were major academicians from leading universities and our programs were fully affiliated with university programs. Within the next five years, six of us retired or resigned from our positions and the seventh was fired two years later.

I had heard that one confrere had brought in a full-time cancer surgeon from Roswell Park. I knew this fellow, and he was a superb technical surgeon. I called my friend and told him, in jest, that he had just sealed his fate. By bringing in a good operating surgeon he would antagonize his staff. We laughed. Within two years he was back in an academic position at a major university and the surgeon he had put on staff had similarly left for another job. As for my teaching credentials, I was made director of surgical education for the department at the medical school. Subsequently, I won the approval of the medical school faculty, and was honored as the best teacher for two consecutive years by the faculty (see Appendix), and also the residents and students.

The quality of the operations performed at this hospital were mostly quite good. I monitored the cases that were done and tried to correct deficiencies when I saw them. As some surgeons aged, we quietly encouraged retirement and taking on a younger partner. The referring doctors knew who the most accomplished doctors were. But quality varies, particularly when difficult advanced cases presented, or in elderly patients. I could not guarantee that all referrals were made in the best interests of the patient. There were hints of fee splitting. Some weak surgeons continued to get into trouble, but usually were able to ask for assistance when needed. Many of my referrals were from former or current colleagues (surgeons), but in the final analysis the patient and family must remain diligent in determining how to reach the most qualified doctors (see Chapter 9).

CHAPTER 7: BACK AT THE UNIVERSITY

Although I was tenured at New Jersey Medical School, I could retain my title and a minimum salary but no guarantee of anything to do. My chief decided to offer a position as director of surgical education.

I loved this challenge, and soon developed a number of changes in the curriculum and expanded the educational program to include scattered lectures and weekly exams. This latter activity was carried out by sending the exams to the students by e-mail, and requiring their responses to be sent to me. I devised a series of clinical problems illustrating important surgical principles and graded the responses. No short-answer questions were used. Although the students could use any reference material they desired, the questions required detailed responses. Then I followed with a lecture by a faculty member (often me) on the same clinical problems, indicating a line of analysis and appropriate solutions. While this seemed like a fertile approach, there were a number of serious problems in the teaching program which I labored to solve. I was rewarded two consecutive years by faculty recognition as the best teacher at the institution, a feat infrequently duplicated by surgeons. In my last year, the senior students honored me by electing me to lead the entry of faculty at the annual graduation ceremony. I also received teaching plaques from the surgical residents.

Teaching at The Medical School

Medicine had changed drastically since my student days.

Reduced hospital stays are required to control costs. This means outpatient work-ups and same-day surgery. While this does not affect and may often improve patient care, it is difficult for students to maintain continuity from initial evaluation to recovery for many diseases. They often see patients for the first time on the operating table, thereby limiting the availability of history-taking and physical examination. They lose the ability to work through diagnostic steps that used to be routine. Furthermore, diagnostic studies have become so technologically advanced that physical diagnosis is often bypassed. The stethoscope has given way to the CAT scan and echocardiogram.

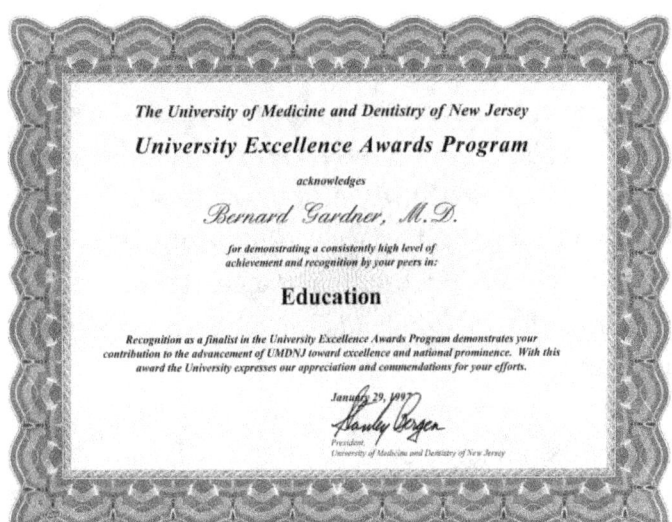

The University of Medicine and Dentistry of New Jersey

University Excellence Awards Program

acknowledges

Bernard Gardner, M.D.

for demonstrating a consistently high level of
achievement and recognition by your peers in:

Education

Recognition as a finalist in the University Excellence Awards Program demonstrates your
contribution to the advancement of UMDNJ toward excellence and national prominence. With this
award the University expresses our appreciation and commendations for your efforts.

January 29, 1997

President,
University of Medicine and Dentistry of New Jersey

I was honored to have been recognized for my contributions to the academic community in 1997 and 1998.

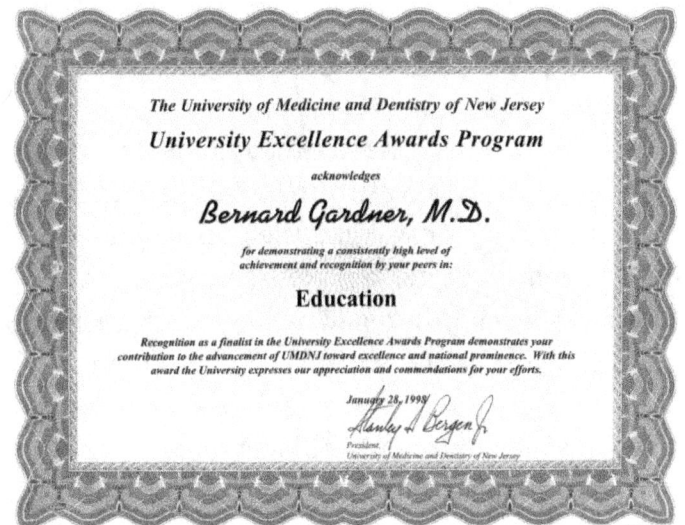

The University of Medicine and Dentistry of New Jersey

University Excellence Awards Program

acknowledges

Bernard Gardner, M.D.

for demonstrating a consistently high level of
achievement and recognition by your peers in:

Education

Recognition as a finalist in the University Excellence Awards Program demonstrates your
contribution to the advancement of UMDNJ toward excellence and national prominence. With this
award the University expresses our appreciation and commendations for your efforts.

January 28, 1998

President,
University of Medicine and Dentistry of New Jersey

As a result, students miss the opportunity to hear thoracic sounds, or important cardiac murmurs that may tip them off to significant diagnostic clues. This is also true on medicine rotations where pneumonia, etc. have become diseases treated without hospitalization. In previous times, a patient with the rales of pneumonia or a heart murmur was auscultated by the four or five students assigned to the service.

The outpatient clinics are the centers for diagnosis, and the patient selection is varied and unpredictable. Training of specialists moved many patients to the community doctors, and rotation of students to doctors' offices is done at some medical schools in order to provide clinical patients for study. This method of teaching is haphazard in the least, depending on the commitment of the busy private practitioner and his/her interest in teaching.

It was my experience that students at our institution lacked expertise in physical examination and often in history taking (the fundamental basis for diagnosis). After my retirement, I found a similar deficiency in many of the young practicing physicians I encountered. Today there are computer programs which analyze symptoms and signs available for practitioners and students, including photos of various conditions. However, there needs to be a commitment by the physician to read the current literature and engage in post-graduate education when available.

There were other problems. In order for faculty to be promoted and receive tenure, it was vital to publish research papers in peer-reviewed journals, and to present at national meetings. Together with the demands of clinical faculty to support the school by earning money in practice, these requirements greatly limit the time available for teaching students. As a result, faculty often shun local lecture assignments and rotations demanding heavy student contact. As a tenured professor, I carried a high patient load and sacrificed research time to provide time for teaching. Younger faculty could not afford to do this.

Students at many medical schools spend their first two years taking basic sciences courses taught by faculty who often have no or little clinical experience. As a result, their lectures are often hard to relate to real patients or clinical situations. Many schools tried to remedy this problem in several ways: One was to introduce clinical medicine in the second year, with a return to some basic science in the third when it might be better integrated with clinical material in the student's mind. Another was to introduce a combined basic science–clinical curriculum in the second-year to run with conferences combining both types of faculty in the hopes that the integration could be made simpler for the student. But problems persisted.

Some teachers are knowledgeable in their subjects but have little experience in how to teach. They may be obtuse in their presentations, which confuse the students. Courses were developed to help these teachers improve their presentations, frequently to no avail. Students often slept through these lectures, and depended on notes which were published and sold by other students. In one department, a noted scholar was lecturing to a single student with a recording machine. He was so upset that at the next opportunity he recorded his lecture and played it to the other machine. The students complained!

Often, faculty who are excellent teachers may not be interested or proficient in research, and cannot be promoted for lack of publications. We had a neuroscientist on our faculty who designed and ran a basic course in neurology which was enormously successful as a teaching instrument. He ran the whole project by himself, and was adored by the students. He was constantly among their choices as best teacher. But, he could not get promoted. He was denied tenure multiple times.

Many medical schools try to obviate this problem by introducing an educational tenure tract designed to protect the outstanding teacher.

Unfortunately, this doesn't always succeed in providing either promotion or tenure. The academic qualifications committees (the ones responsible for recommending promotion and tenure), usually composed of noted researchers, always concentrate on publications and peer recognition from faculty at other institutions. Since some of these excellent teachers often do not publish or present at meetings, they are unrecognized by outside faculty. In our institution the teaching faculty and the students knew who they were, but failed to convince the administration of their value.

Young faculty recognize the problem and when time is precious, teaching is sacrificed.

Students soon learn that grades depend upon performance on exams. As a result, textbooks are often sacrificed for exam review books in all subjects. The in-depth analysis of disease is often replaced by a series of questions and answers that could be memorized, and likely to appear in some form on future examinations. A need for patients, whom the students can study, necessitates rotations to large community (teaching) hospitals. In these institutions, the teaching is markedly irregular depending on the personal dedication of individual practitioners. Evaluations of the students are equally spotty. Students who were interested in library time to study were generally not appreciated on surgical services. As a result, those of us responsible for final grades depended on standardized examinations to even out the evaluations. Back to the review books for the students.

There was a lack of coordination in teaching, which in my opinion resulted in an inferior graduate. A lot of this was the result of entrenched disciplines (departments) who refused to yield teaching time to those who were better able to present the requisite material, correlated with clinical patient presentations. For example, the function of the GI tract as presented by the physiology department was far removed from the actual patient diseases, as seen from the point of view of a medical gastroenterologist.

We tried to develop correlation clinics to combine the physiology, biochemistry, pathology and anatomy with clinical patient material, but this was hampered by individual departments' entrenched teaching time, which was defended because any cut might result in fewer faculty lines being required (hence a reduction in that department's budget and influence).

What made the situation even worse was that the obvious faculty to teach and correlate all this material for the students were the clinicians.

Many physicians dealing with the GI diseases, for example, are involved with basic and clinical research, and usually thoroughly familiar with the current literature. They are better able to correlate the physiology, pathology, etc. of these diseases, combined with diagnosis and treatment, and present the material so that it makes sense to the student. Basic science faculty members often have not experienced how physiologic derangements present clinically, thereby missing a golden opportunity to impress valuable information on the student. The same is true for our nephrologists and transplant surgeons to teach about renal physiology, or cardiologists and heart surgeons to teach about heart function etc., etc.

But, many clinicians are not likely to spend time teaching students, as noted previously. Their time is absorbed by the need to earn money in practice, and do research for promotion, and often with resident teaching taking a priority position when any time was left over. When I tried to establish clinical correlation courses and to engage clinical faculty in teaching basic material, clinical and physical examination, I could not regularly count on them. It wasn't their fault. Remember that funding for the medical school often depends on grant procurement and earnings from private practice. It is a system that guarantees that students will get short shrift.

I don't mean to be depressing. There is a load of teaching that goes on, often by dedicated faculty members. The questions of effectiveness persist. The technical aspects of medicine and the burgeoning of scientific data require a re-examination of the system. At present, the development of a first-rate physician is left to residency programs. Having dealt with residents over the years, I would modify that even further. It depends clearly on the basic makeup of the resident (and subsequently the physician), and his/her dedication to continued learning and study. This has got to be a very spotty system in spite of a series of in-service examinations that residents are required to take. As a result, the quality of medical care is spread over such a wide spectrum of knowledge and performance, assuring that the patient better be aware of who is providing treatment.

Much of the preparation for clinical practice is left to post-residency fellowships.

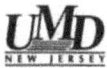

NEW JERSEY MEDICAL SCHOOL

Office of the Dean
Phone: (973) 972-4538
Fax: (973) 972-7104
http://www.umdnj.edu/njmsweb/

185 South Orange Avenue
University Heights
Newark, NJ 07103-2714

April 5, 2000

Bernard Gardner, M.D.
Professor of Surgery
c/o 232 Mountainview Drive
Mahwah, New Jersey 07430

Bernie

Dear Dr. Gardner:

As you know, the Class of 2000 wishes to honor you at the UMDNJ-New Jersey Medical School Convocation by requesting you be the Gonfalon Bearer. You would lead the Class of 2000 in the processional and carry the gonfalon. Convocation is scheduled for Sunday, May 21, 2000, at 1:00 p.m.

Ms. Linda Reich, of my office, has confirmed that you are willing to be the Gonfalon Bearer, and that you are making arrangements to order your academic attire. Please be assured that within the next few weeks, my office will provide you with further details.

Congratulations on being selected by the students for this honor!

Sincerely,

Tony

Anthony J. Garro, Ph.D.
Vice Dean
Chairman, Convocation Committee

c: Ruy V. Lourenço, M.D., Dean
Linda C. Reich, M.B.A., Director of Special Projects
Edwin A. Deitch, M.D., Chair, Surgery

University of Medicine & Dentistry of New Jersey

A token of appreciation from my students that touched me deeply.

I learned most of patient diagnosis and treatment at a patient bedside during my residency years.

Can these problems be solved? Absolutely! While there is much variation among medical schools, common problems exist. I was once on an NIH committee to give teaching grants to universities. We site-visited a major Ivy League institution. The faculty for the grant was composed of world-renowned specialists. Part of the visit was spent interviewing the students for whom the grant was intended. They confided that they rarely or ever had contact with these prestigious faculty members. It was clear that the teaching was successful, because the caliber of the students was so high that they were fully capable of self-instruction using the current literature.

Medical schools are rigorously evaluated on a regular basis in order to maintain accreditation. Often, several days are devoted to these activities when disinterested faculty from other schools interview students, local faculty and administrators, as well as reviewing curricula documentation. All aspects of the teaching programs are reviewed, to be certain that minimum standards are met. No local faculty member or student is likely to discuss any curricular shortcomings involving his own school. What is lacking in these reviews, in my opinion, is a thorough evaluation of the students' knowledge base over several hours of questioning. When I was in charge of fellowship certification for the Society of Surgical Oncology, such sessions with the fellows were enlightening in revealing the true value of the described teaching sessions. I don't mean to demean the efforts of reviewers, or lower the value of board exams given to certify physicians, but rather to help pinpoint the problems so medical school deans would have ammunition to make necessary changes.

I have been retired for some years and have not recently reviewed programs at many medical schools. I am sure that many improvements may have been made. Physical diagnosis is supplemented by computer programs, and diagnostic criteria can be accumulated by similar programs.

The following observations might lead to some solutions:

Students are best at evaluating their peers. This has been repeatedly demonstrated. Some schools provide tutors from the ranks of fourth year students.

Residents often use the year following completion of the residency program to study for their boards while taking time off from practice (sometimes in a faculty position or fellowship). They are uniquely qualified to teach students and young residents. Every medical school should provide one-year post-residency teaching fellowships with sufficient reimbursement to make them competitive. The requirements should include multiple hours of teaching physical examination and clinical problem solving, etc. in their specialty. Board examinations, for which these residents are preparing, often test basic science knowledge, guaranteeing that these residents are up-to-date. This information can be imparted to students and PGY 1 and 2 residents in a clinical setting.

Combined clinical-basic science courses in the third (or second) year should have independent departmental status to hire basic scientists and clinicians as faculty (their own budgets). These courses should have a curriculum independent of interference by other departments in the medical school. Basic scientists should be encouraged to attend clinical rounds and conferences.

The fourth year of medical school should be better controlled. Presently, some students may use the time to audition for residency positions. The educational value of the electives is often suspect with little involvement of the home institution. Teaching is extremely variable. One or two-week sub-specialty rotations should be abandoned. Busy emergency rooms provide excellent teaching opportunities.

Teaching of diseases of the eyes, ears, etc. should be incorporated into the physical diagnosis courses in earlier years. One-month sub-internships can be offered as electives in the fourth year, with strict teaching and grading requirements. Faculty members at the home institution should be charged with strict evaluation of all electives wherever they may be located.

Standardized tests involving physical diagnosis and critical thinking should be given in the fourth year, utilizing standard patients (hired actors or patients). Faculty often cannot muster the time to conduct these tests when the class exceeds a hundred students. With medical classes of that size, it is necessary for the administration to take a serious look at full-time teaching faculty. After all, why does a medical school exist if its primary function is not teaching medical students?

In this day and age of physician and surgical assistants, I have noted that many of these individuals are better-fitted to handle clinical problems, including diagnosis and treatment, than our fourth-year medical students and often our PGY 1 and 2 residents. These individuals can make excellent teachers at the bedside.

Most importantly, the supervision and design of the teaching program and design of its courses must be given to an independent, multi-disciplinary committee of senior faculty. For example, a course on heart disease should involve both clinicians and basic scientists.

Teaching professionals should be hired and evaluated by this committee.

Clinical faculty at affiliated hospitals must be willing to spend one full day weekly for scheduled rotations with students, in order to maintain their faculty appointments. Students are entitled to bedside teaching and individual review of their history and physical examination write-ups. Rotating students provides help and prestige for these clinicians. In this day of practice groups, such teaching assignments should be possible. Many (in some areas, most) patients who would become teaching subjects are located in affiliated hospitals.

On a serious note: A close friend recently called to ask my advice concerning his wife, who was starting pre-operative chemotherapy for a locally advanced breast cancer. She had been followed for a year after complaining about a breast mass and having two "negative" mammograms. Clearly, the family practitioner either forgot or was never told that the only way to diagnose a palpable breast mass exactly is by biopsy. His clinical examination skills were faulty. The radiologist never examined the patient. To my mind this is often a failure at the medical school level.

I strongly apologize for any of my views which may have been adjudicated since I left academia some years ago. This book is a look back at teaching and practice of medicine in previous years. My recent contacts with doctors, however, point to continuing problems that may require attention.

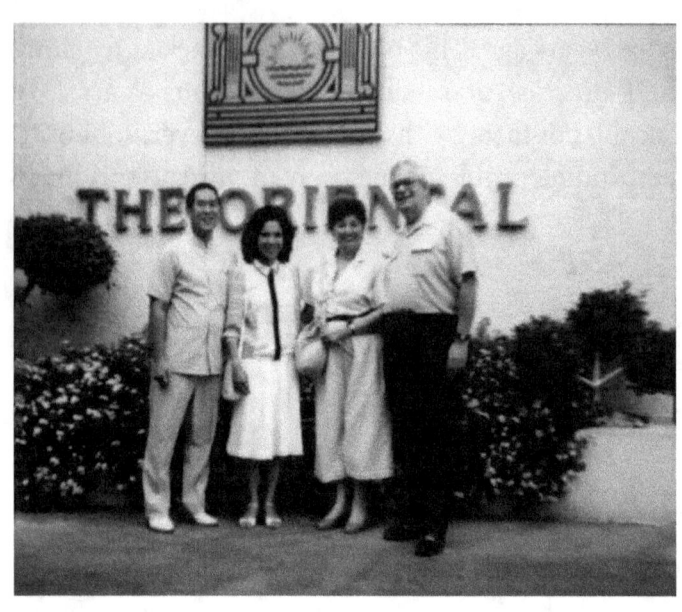

With colleagues in Thailand

CHAPTER 8: EXTRACURRICULAR ACTIVITIES

I mentioned in previous sections that we ran an animal lab at the medical school. Early publications revolved around basic science questions involving calcium metabolism, tumor growth and spread, the activity of cell surface in solutions, leading to biliary tract studies and stone formation. In later years, we published many articles on clinical management. All told, over 170 peer-reviewed papers and articles were published, and multiple presentations here and abroad on visiting professorships. The appendix includes a selection of published papers.

Among the activities that consumed the most time were three edited textbooks. One, Basic Surgery, edited by two other well-known surgeons and myself, went into five editions. It was an unusual teaching system which taught surgery according to the way patients presented clinically, rather than according to standard disease categories. For example, there were chapters on GI bleeding, diarrhea, abdominal pain and other symptoms which covered the physiology of these conditions and the diagnostic steps and subsequent management. There were no chapters on diseases of the colon, etc. Those students who used the book were delighted with this method of presentation.

The other books were one on trauma surgery and a short book on cancer surgery, which covered many of the operative techniques we developed on our tumor service with a young head and neck surgeon, Tony Alfonso, and Horace Herbsman, the former trauma specialist.

I received a letter from India inviting me to speak at a cancer seminar with other oncologists. Arrangements were handled by an Indian group, which included airfare, registration at a fine hotel, meals and a two-day safari ordered through Cooks travel agency in London. It turned out to be a memorable event.

We landed in Delhi at 11 p.m. in this huge airport with monkeys swinging from many rafters. Men grabbed my luggage, offering to carry the bags for a tip. We held on, stopping at a booth with an English-speaking person. We were directed out of a door along an open corridor, and told that there was an uprising going on. The streets were manned by soldiers with machine guns. We found the taxi booth with our driver. Getting into an old black Mercedes with all the red panel lights flashing. There were cows walking the streets.

I felt we were in a James Bond film but without the script.

We arrived at our hotel, an American luxury hotel, at which we had a suite with full bar and snacks, all free. Trouble was, we had a plane to catch at 10 a.m. Back in the airport, the plane finally took off to Bangalore (our destination) at 1 p.m.

In Bangalore, there were representatives of our hotel present to carry our luggage and load us in a bus to our hotel. As we waited at a traffic light, I noticed a svelte man in a three-piece dark grey suit and with an attaché case, which he carefully placed on the corner sidewalk and promptly started to urinate. Welcome to Bangalore!

We stayed at a government-run hotel with first-class rooms, and all meals were served at an extensive buffet in the gardens.

My lectures were heavily attended. I noticed many doctors shaking their heads back and forth. I felt depressed. When I returned to my room, Joan had hired a car and driver to take us on a day trip to a regional castle. She said that when she asked for a car, the clerk shook his head from side to side, and that meant it was ok. I was a hit and didn't know it.

One Indian surgeon stopped to ask me about a patient he had with liver metastases from a colon cancer. As I began to describe how to proceed with a liver resection, he stopped me. He just wanted to know what drugs I would use to provide pain relief. Very sad.

Joan and I were invited to a grand dinner at the palatial home of the governor of Bangalore. Later, we were notified that Cooks Travel had given our lodge rooms to a group from National Geographic.

I mentioned this to one of our hosts, and a day later we were rebooked in the lodge and the other group were placed in tents. When I returned to my hotel after the safari, I noticed that a pair of expensive jade cuff links were missing. I reported it at the hotel and we saw police in the halls on several occasions, but the cuff links were still missing. Six months later, I received a package from India which contained my jewelry with a note that they were found under the bed. Either they were very slow in cleaning the room, or somebody was caught when trying to sell them.

For many years there was a well-known society, known as the James Ewing Society, made up of graduates from the training programs at Memorial Sloan Kettering Hospital in New York. The members felt that the society needed a broader base of surgeons, and they decided to take other qualified members. I was one of the earliest surgeons asked to join this new society, to be known as "The Society of Surgical Oncology, formerly the James Ewing Society." In later years it dropped the latter designation, and became The Society of Surgical Oncology. In addition to yearly presentations of scientific papers, they supported fellowship programs at other major institutions to help develop the specialty One day the president of the society asked me to take over these fellowship programs and develop a curriculum for them, and to assess the teaching programs, and to be sure that they were producing adequately- trained surgeons who would become future members of the society. This task involved me and one of the other member of my committee visiting every program (there were about ten) for two days each, for total review of the teaching and experience of the fellows. All of the department chairmen we visited were cooperative, and where possible very helpful in instituting our recommendations, even though some of the programs were dropped from approval by the society. I mention this to indicate that subsequently, over the years, I became secretary, admissions chairman, and in 1994 president of the society (at the time having 1200 members). The presidential meeting was superb, involving an annual speech which I gave to review the development of surgical oncology as a specialty. We stayed in a huge suite with my wife and three children. I arranged for many important guest speakers, and two special parties for past presidents and special guest invitees, many of whom had been my students.

I held many other offices in different societies, but this was special, having watched its growth from its earliest years. Today the society is much larger, and the fellowship programs have increased and include special breast cancer fellowships. If a cancer patient is referred to a member of the society for operation, he (she) will be in good hands. I have avoided stressing clinical cases and operations in this book, in spite of some spectacular cases that I managed. Any dedicated cancer surgeon could duplicate some of those procedures.

CHAPTER 9: A SUMMARY OF WHAT PATIENTS NEED TO KNOW

You may need an operation for one of many reasons.

Elective Procedures:
You have chronic pain in hip, knee, shoulder back etc. You have exhausted non-operative treatment such as rest, injections in the back or involved joint, without adequate relief. Your family doctor has recommended evaluation by a surgeon and made the referral, or several of your neighbors or friends may have had a successful procedure by a surgeon, or there is a hospital that specializes in the procedure you require. The operation is commonly performed with new techniques involving smaller incisions and new prosthetic material and minimal rehabilitation. The operation may involve a wait, without danger, of days, weeks or months, depending on the surgeon's schedule.

In this category I would include hernia, some peripheral vein or artery surgery or a dermatologic procedure, although some of these may have to be done more propitiously. Again, it is important to choose a surgeon who specializes in these procedures.

Many of these operations will be performed as an outpatient (same day surgery). Your surgeon (his staff) may contact your family doctor to determine if any of your medical problems or medications could interfere with a smooth surgical outcome, or your doctor may have sent a report on his own. The surgical offices will have you fill out a detailed medical history and list of medications. You will be scheduled for routine laboratory tests and a chest x-ray. If you are having general anesthesia, you should undergo an anesthesia evaluation in the hospital. There may be a direct contact with an anesthesiologist if you are over 60 or have a history of cardiac or pulmonary disease or are taking or have intolerance for certain medications.

Tips for Choosing a Good Doctor

In my retirement community I have been frequently asked for referral suggestions. If I cannot evaluate the local surgeons, I will often send patients to major institutions or specialty hospitals where I am confident of the experience and quality of the care. I am sometimes cognizant of results of surgery in members of my community, whether good or bad. My family doctor works in a hospital-based group, and will make recommendations honestly. He often will tell me that so-and-so is a whiz at a certain procedure, but I have no qualms about sending a patient to a university hospital, where many advanced cases are. treated

For patients facing with a prospective operation, my experiences led to several important observations.

Choosing a surgeon is more important than choosing a hospital. The expertise of the surgeon is most valuable. I have commented on how to evaluate a hospital in other sections, but even the best of hospitals may have surgeons with different experiences on staff.

Ask your surgeon questions at length about his training and experiences, mortality rate, the availability of good anesthesiologists and qualified consultants if something goes wrong and who covers him if he is not available. If he rebels at these questions, get another surgeon. His ego should not get in the way of his consideration for you.

Chances are that your family physician has recommended a surgeon. Why? What does he know about her qualifications?

Would he recommend that surgeon for his spouse or parents?

The surgeon will often choose the anesthesiologist or at least consult with him (her). It is vital in extensive operations, or those in elderly patients, that the surgeon keep track of what is happening to avoid complications.

Overhydration or use of narcotics in the elderly can negate the results of good surgery. I often did operations in some high-risk patients under local anesthesia to avoid complications. In many institutions, nurse anesthetists will give anesthesia, but they should be monitored by physicians. Be careful if one physician is monitoring multiple rooms, as he/she may not be available in an emergency. (Sometimes, rarely, the nurse will be more or as capable as the physician assigned. Your surgeon will know and should exert his responsibility to be certain that all is well.)

Your visit with the surgeon is the time to ask questions. Is there danger of mortality with the procedure? (There is no such thing as a simple operation.) What are his results? Who will give anesthesia, a boarded anesthesiologist or a nurse anesthetist? Will he or she be supervised? How many procedures will the supervising anesthesiologist be covering at the same time? (I hope not more than two.) If the surgeon is reticent or annoyed about answering questions such as these, use your judgment about continuing. If you are over 70, it is important to have an experienced anesthesiologist available since your reaction to some narcotics or sedatives may be very different from that of younger patients.

Semi-Elective Procedures

Some diseases require an operation after a period of non-operative treatment or a failure of non-operative treatment. Previous diagnostic studies have indicated an inflammation of the gallbladder or colon, and operation is recommended. Your family doctor has selected a surgical consultant who recommends operation. There may be many examples of other conditions falling into this category. Various nodules, thyroid or breast lumps are some examples. Admission to the hospital is often recommended, particularly if a major body cavity (abdomen or thorax) will be entered.

The preoperative routine is similar to the one described. Additionally, specialty consultation (cardiologic or infectious disease) may be sought.

This may indicate that you have a more serious condition and will demand more attention on you or your family member's part. The surgeon's experience and occasionally special training should be checked.

An Aside: I once had dinner with a member of the New York board of Regents, a group responsible for the licensing of physicians. I asked him why, when a doctor completes his (her) internship and passes the state board exam, he/she is licensed to practice medicine and surgery.

His answer was that if I would come and practice in upstate rural New York, he would change the rule. Clearly patients, particularly in underserved areas, are at the mercy of the available services. Travel to other hospitals may not be possible for some families. Surgery may be legally performed by a doctor who has no or minimal surgical training.

Some hospitals specialize in various disciplines: children's, orthopedic, cancer, are a few examples. Others are known for their advanced training: Mayo Clinic, Cleveland Clinic, most major university hospitals. Since many of their trainees end up practicing in community hospitals, there is often little need to travel to these institutions unless you cannot find the expertise you are seeking, or prefer more experienced surgeons. Often, a large community hospital will train residents and provide advanced fellowship training or develop special areas of expertise (i.e. joint replacement, open heart surgery, etc.) and your family physician should be aware of this.

Remember: Some surgeons will pass on patients who are poor risks to avoid increasing their mortality rates.

Levels of Training:
It may be confusing, when arriving in a hospital, as to the large number of persons involved in your

care. Trained nurses are in short supply throughout the U.S. (actually world-wide).

Registered nurses take 2 to 4 years of post-graduate study and pass an exam in most states. They will usually serve as the head nurse on the ward. They also serve as specialty nurses in ICUs or special cardiac units and most ERs and ORs. They make rounds, administer medications and see that doctors' orders are carried out. They are also responsible for seeing that detailed notes are charted, among other major duties.

These nurses are assisted by other nurses, LPNs (licensed practical nurses), assistant nurses, trainees, etc. who carry out other direct-patient activities, from monitoring vital signs to assisting patients to walk or go to the bathroom.

Multiple techs are available to start IVs, draw lab bloods, administer pulmonary treatments and lower level personnel to clean rooms, and transport patients.

Nurse Practitioners have special additional training. They are licensed to see patients under a doctor's supervision and prescribe certain medications. They do complete patient examinations, and are useful in some acute care facilities. A few state medical societies resist their invasion of medical care. (My prediction is that they will be useful as primary care givers due to a shortage of family physicians, or in communities where doctors don't want to practice.)

Doctors and Other Medical Professionals

House Doctors are sometimes hired by hospitals to provide direct inpatient care. They are general practitioners or occasionally older or foreign-trained specialists not in active practice. They handle all emergency calls from many areas of the hospital and emergency admissions from the ER. This allows private doctors to be free to tend to their office practices.

Specialists are available on call for problems when needed.

Fellows: Post-residency specialty training programs are located in some larger hospitals. Examples are joint replacement, microsurgery, vascular surgery, cardiology, and many others. The fellow will examine you after identifying himself, and consult with your admitting doctor. These are usually highly-trained (male or female) doctors planning to enter the specialty.

Residents: These are doctors who are rotating through the discipline that brought you to the hospital. They may be at various levels of training, but will examine you prior to your procedure and consult with your surgeon. They are responsible for putting a detailed history and physical examination on the chart. When present, they are the ones called first in an emergency at night or post op, and will make daily rounds on all assigned patients.

They usually take the place of house doctors.

Physician Assistants: These are non-doctors who have two or three years of post-graduate training and are licensed by the state. I have always found them to be diligent and dedicated, and have encouraged them to participate in the care of patients. (They are similar to the medical techs found in the military who carry out multiple procedures.) They are usually knowledgeable about your condition and its treatment.

Medical Students: Don't be afraid! You are safer being seen by multiple persons in hospitals than a single doctor. The doctor dealing with students had better be up-to-date on the current medical literature. This is better than a surgeon who reports his results to nobody. I have seen multiple instances where a diligent medical student has found important elements on history or physical exam that might influence treatment.

Emergency Procedures

I am excluding trauma from this book. Many states have designated trauma units, levels 1 to 3, sometimes associated with an air transport service and specially-trained surgeons. Home injuries are often treated at local hospital ERs after 911 medical transport. You will be treated by doctors at that ER to which you are transported.

It's no use calling your local doctor. You will be directed to call 911.

Most ERs are manned by general practitioners or doctors who have trained in emergency medicine residencies, are qualified and have joined groups which work under contract to a hospital. ASK!

Significant delays may occur due to numbers of patients in the unit, or inadequate coverage, or rarely, lack of empty beds. Hospitals advertise waiting periods in minutes, but this usually refers to intake data, not time to see a doctor, which could be exasperatingly long.

There has been a rise in availability of walk-in clinics (urgent care centers), which are open for long hours, with lower waiting times, but you need to have appropriate insurance coverage or cash on hand. They may be exceedingly expensive (as are ERs) for uninsured patients, and they are usually not set up for surgical emergencies.

I have always felt that ER waiting times are much reduced if you are brought in on a gurney by EMTs, rather than to drive over and walk in.

Two conditions that result in rapid treatment (by necessity) are chest pain or stroke symptoms, because results of treatment for strokes or myocardial infarction are directly related to the speed with which treatment is initiated. Injuries due to falls at home may be associated with either of these conditions. Resulting injuries may require orthopedic consultation or management. Usually a CAT scan of the head is done in patients who fell, to avoid missing an associated intracranial injury (bleeding).

When you have an acute surgical emergency presenting with abdominal pain, your results will depend on the rapidity of diagnosis, the knowledge of the ER doctor, the availability of surgical consultation and sometimes the quality and experience of the consultant. X-rays, CAT scans and laboratory analysis are available in the ER of most hospitals, but the hands and brain of the ER doctor is most valuable. Elderly or diabetic patients require the most meticulous evaluation, because physical signs and symptoms could be masked or unreliable in these patients. Delay in diagnosis is rampant in some ERs and accounts for a large number of malpractice suits. It may help to leave a message with your family doctor as to where you are and why.

If an operation is necessary, the same rules hold for the surgeon to confer with the patient and family. Consultations may be necessary but everything, including workup is expedited. Preoperative IV or blood stabilization may be required.

The Elderly Patient

I want to emphasize that no patient should be denied a necessary operation based on age alone. Later in my career, we published an evaluation of 375 patients over the age of 80 who underwent major operations. Mortality was related to the stage of disease and not age. Patients who saw regular physicians and were operated upon electively did as well or better than younger patients. Only those admitted as emergencies had high mortality rates. One of our patients celebrated her 100th birthday in the hospital, post-colectomy for cancer. This was reported in a local daily newspaper.

Sometimes the approach may be altered. I have operated many times under local anesthesia to perform a life-saving temporary procedure on older patients, or those with serious diseases who face a high mortality for operation under general anesthesia. Often, after stabilization, at a later time, a definitive procedure can be safely completed days or weeks later. This may be preferred occasionally in younger patients. I have performed major resections (mastectomy) under local anesthesia and IV sedation in patients with severe heart disease, who were felt by anesthesiologists to be a major risk for general anesthesia.

This book is not meant as a political treatise, but it would not be complete without noting the detrimental effects of lack of adequate medical insurance on patients' prospects for survival from serious diseases. When the only choice for treatment is the emergency room, mortality is always higher for emergency operations and for patients with inadequate routine care. I am not including morbidity due to the effects of financial ruin from the high costs of medical care.

Patients with Advanced Disease

Dealing with patients who have advanced disease or cancer has occurred multiple times in my experience. On some occasions, patients referred by other surgeons because of advanced or recurrent disease have undergone re-operation, and after resection have been cancer free. This is particularly true with colon cancer, some cases of biliary cancer, and occasional cases of stage 3 breast cancer. (There are other similar cases reported by other surgical oncologists.) On occasion, supplemental treatment with radiation or chemotherapy is required.

Rarely cancer, usually associated with older patients, may occur in young adults or children. I've treated rectal cancer in a 13-year-old girl and another with fibrosarcoma of the abdominal wall, and a fourteen-year-old with melanoma in the head and neck area, and another with pancreatic cancer. *Among the tragic cases I've had was a newly-married 20-year-old Hispanic boy we operated upon for an acute abdominal condition. We found an abdomen filled with studded growths throughout, which I misdiagnosed as tuberculosis at first. A biopsy showed adenocarcinoma. Neither he nor his 19-year-old new wife or his mother spoke English. We had to use a person who could communicate in Spanish to explain the condition.*

Wherever I practiced, I set up a tumor board made up of hematologists, medical oncologists, surgeons and radiologists and assorted nurses and any professional interested in cancer management. We encouraged practitioners to present their cancer patients, before treatment, for review and discussion at these weekly sessions. Everyone contributed their expertise and we discussed planned treatment. There were differences of opinion in some cases, but usually a consensus was reached and usually carried out. In my opinion, this should be available in every hospital where cancer patients are treated, even if it is necessary to reach for outside experts. While it is not necessary for routine cases, many times problems appear that require discussion or opinions of other specialties to improve management.

If you or a family member is diagnosed with cancer, be certain to contact an expert to get your treatment on the right track. Get a second opinion if an operation is necessary, and you may even need to confirm the pathologic diagnosis. Usually the first thing the consulting surgeon does is to have the pathology slides re-evaluated by his chosen pathologist. If necessary, he/she will arrange consultation with medical or radiation oncologists.

The wife of a friend was scheduled to start chemotherapy for multiple myeloma (a tumor of the bone marrow,) based on a lesion in a rib and a needle aspiration bone biopsy diagnosed by a local pathologist. I discussed the possibility of seeing an oncologist at our local cancer hospital for a second opinion. A direct rib biopsy was performed, removing a segment of bone. Studies found it was a benign lesion and not cancerous.

There are often times when no treatment is available which will prolong the life of a cancer patient. As I indicated above, I always was honest with the patient and at least one member of the family. I never believed that hiding facts of the condition from the patient would be fruitful, and therefore I avoided it. Today, the use of hospice care and end-of-life counseling plays a large role in management. There are palliative care specialists available in many hospitals and home hospice care. The use of pain killers are well- managed by these experts.

In previous times, doctors and nurses carried this out. No family ever asked me to help a patient die, but I made certain that the patient in this condition was pain-free, and no one was ordering unnecessary tests. I believed that a patient with an endearing family would best be allowed to die at home. Home care nurses and home hospice are often available to ease the transition.

Experimental Treatments

The National Institutes of Health (NIH) funds multiple national studies of treatment of a large number of cancers. These are carried out at local institutions under protocols that are rigidly followed to guarantee reproducible results. These treatments include a control group, along with the experimental (new treatment) group which provides the highest level of evidence that the results are reliable.

I participated as an early member of the NSABP, which was responsible for proving the success of breast preservation procedures in providing cures for many patients with breast cancer. The group eventually moved on to the use of chemotherapy in breast and colon cancer. Many such groups are currently evaluating treatments for just about every type and location of cancer. A well-trained oncologist will know about these studies, and can recommend that a patient might want to enter such a study. The control group is always treated by the best available current treatment, and no charges are made for follow-up and use of experimental drugs or other experimental treatment.

There are numerous unproven homeopathic medications or drugs suggested by friends, family or poorly-trained doctors. Many of these are discussed in literature obtainable from the National Cancer Institute of the NIH. I have never dismissed a patient who traveled to Lourdes or used some local drugs to treat his (her) cancer, but usually recommended a treatment that I thought might be more efficacious.

Do Doctors Always Agree?

If you go to a medical conference you would find about as much agreement as you might find in the Israeli Knesset in passing a law on immigration. Remember the old story about the guy who was just informed that he had two months to live. The doctor asked if there was anything he wanted.

"I would like a second opinion," he said.

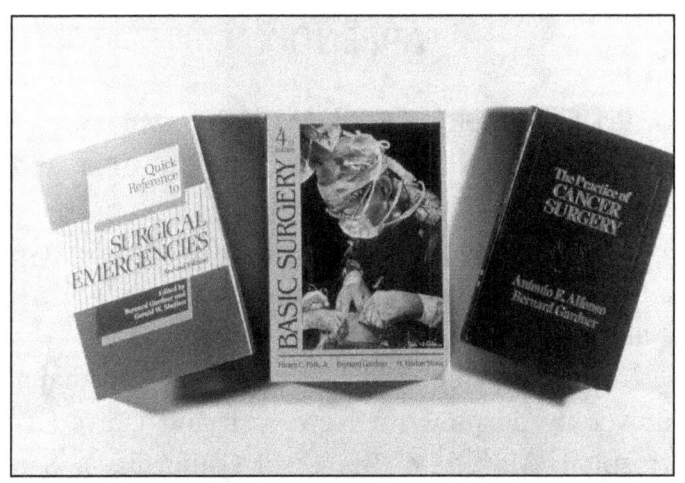

Some of the medical texts written by Dr. Gardner

APPENDIX

Brief biography of Bernard Gardner M.D.

Graduated NYU undergraduate in 1952 and Medical School in 1956.

Retired as a major in the U. S. Air Force Reserve and served as a lieutenant colonel in the New York National Guard.

Trained on the surgical services at two major university hospitals in New York and University Hospital (Moffitt) of the U. of California in San Francisco. He began my academic career at SUNY Downstate in New York and rose to full professor and director of the surgical oncology service. Awarded a John and Mary Markle scholarship in academic medicine in 1968 (similar to a Rhodes or Fulbright scholarship). Chairman of Surgery at a New Jersey hospital (now the 6th largest voluntary hospital in the US) and completed his career as professor and director of surgical education at the New Jersey Medical School (UMDNJ).

His career spanned 35 years, during which he published over 170 peer-reviewed papers and abstracts, over 50 textbook chapters, and co-edited three different textbooks of surgery. His "Basic Surgery" reached five editions. His research was funded by a large number of federal and foundation grants.

Dr. Gardner served as an officer or president of numerous medical and surgical societies, and as chairman of many state and national committees and study sections of the NIH. He served on the boards of three major foundations, including the Research Foundation of the State University of New York, which reports directly to the chancellor. He was president of the prestigious Society of Surgical Oncology, and has been an invited visiting professor at many U.S. institutions and in Europe and Asia. He was promoted to professor emeritus in surgery upon retirement.

Since retirement to Venice with his wife Joan, he has self-published books and five plays. Some of his plays were performed at his golf club by an amateur group to sellout audiences. Tickets were not sold, and the actors received no compensation. Joan and Dr. Gardner have children scattered in New York state, Thailand and two daughters in Florida, plus five grandchildren and three great grandchildren,

He was recently accepted for inclusion in the 2011 edition of "Who's Who in the World," and received a Lifetime Achievement Award from Who's Who.

(The non-medical book titles: "The Value of Corruption in a Democratic Society" by A. Professor; "Living with the Geckos" by Dr. Gardner, his daughter and son-in-law, and "Nuggets–Five Plays" by B. Gardner)

SELECTED ARTICLES

Chosen to illustrate some activities related to surgical oncology

Gardner, B. and Gordan,G.S.: Does urinary calcium reflect growth or regression of disseminated breast cancer? Journal of Clinical Endocrinology and Metababolism, 1962; 22: 627-630.

Gardner, B., Dollinger, M., Silen, W., Back, N. and O'Reilly, S.: Studies in the carcinoid syndrome: Its relation to serotonin, bradykinin, and histamine. Surgery 1967; 62: 362-365.

Gardner, B. The relation between serum calcium and tumor metastases. S.G.&O.1969;128: 369-374.

Gardner, B., Kottmeier, P. and Harshaw, D.: A modified and one-stage pull-through operation for carcinoma or prolapse of the rectum. S.G.&O. 1973; 136:94-99.

Lim, B., Gardner, B., Dennis, C. and Newman, J.: Analysis of survival versus patient and doctor delay in treatment in gastrointestinal cancer. American Journal of Surgery, 1974; 127: 210-214.

Gardner, B., Shin, H. and Alfonso, A.: Repair of large chest wall defects using pedicle flaps. Amer. Jour. Surg. 1976; 132: 406. (This was a subject of a film for the American College of Surgery.)

Gardner, B., Bivona, J., Alfonso, A. and Herbsman, H.: Major surgery in Jehovah's Witnesses: New York State Jour. Med. 1976; 76:5.

Gardner, B., Dotan, J., Shaikh, L., Feldman, J., Herbsman, H., Alfonso, A. and Iyers, S.: The influence of age on survival of adult patients with colon cancer. Surg. Gyn & Obs. 1981; 53: 366-368.

Gardner, B.: The rationale for liver resection for metastatic colon carcinoma. J. Med. Soc. of NJ 1985; 82: 306-308.

Gardner, B.: Five-year survival after extended resection of colon cancer. Jour. Surg. Oncology 1987; 34: 258-261.

Gardner, B.: Resection of proximal bile duct cancer involving the hepatic artery with five-year survival. NJ Med 1989: 86,10: 797-799.

Gardner, B., Rauscher, G. and Palasti, S.: The use of the rotation flap for forehead defects: Contemporary Surg. 1990; 2: 26-29.

Gardner, B. and Palasti, S.: Comparison of hospital costs and morbidity between octogenarians and other patients undergoing general surgery operations: S.G.&O 1990; vol. 171,10: 299-304.

Gardner, B.: Letter to the editor, "Training in Surgical Oncology," J. Surg. Oncol. 1990: 43:1

Gardner, B., Bender, S. and Praeger, P.: Hepatic caudate lobe and partial vena cava resection using a

Gott shunt for retro-hepatic caval bypass. J. Surg. Oncol. 1992; 50: 267-269.

Gardner, B. and Bland, K.: Practice guidelines for major cancer sites. Society of Surgical Oncology. Compiled from Oncology, June, July, August and September 1997 vol. II, numbers 6,7,8 and 9.

I thank all my devoted and efficient secretaries who did much to help me in each of my assignments.

Two Letters

During the course of my career, my best memories are of the warm relations I had with patients who trusted me with their lives. Below are two letters I treasure that illustrate those kinds of relationships.

November 13, 1999

Dear Dr. Gardner,

I am writing concerning your retirement because I can't express myself in words of how I feel concerning you leaving. You know it is very hard on me, bringing many emotions such as fear, sadness, stress, tears, panic, anxiety, depression and questions with no answers. I never expected to live to see you retire. Why! I don't know.

However, you are human and you must have some time in your life to do the things you have long put off because of your special call to science and medicine. I thank God that you will have time to relax and enjoy the rest of your life. I doubt seriously that you will do just that, because you put, your whole self into your profession and I know one day you are just going to think about the poor little old lady me (Mary) and so many others like me, then start the process of getting busy researching science and medicine to conquer that monster cancer.

I believe there was a reason I had to meet such a dedicated, committed stern, caring, gentle doctor as you. When I came to you nearly ten years ago I was a basket case, in a stage of my lie that only the Supreme Being knew the absolute. According to man's study and outcome there is no way I should be alive and well this day, but "it's amazing" as you would say to me. What's good about this Amazing Grace is, that you were part of it. You must be one special doctor not only on earth but also in heaven.

I know and you know that, I am a miracle and that we are thankful for this miracle. There are three parts to me, my body, soul/mind and spirit and my spirit is totally dedicated to God, my soul/my mind is here and in heaven, my body is here. You help so much with my body and soul/mind (psychological being) all that you had control and could do. I believe with all my heart that you took care of me to the best of your abilities. Now! Who will take your place in my life of health...No one! God will just have to help me adjust (smile). Losing a dear friend in the medical field is not easy.

After you operated on me I came home and I was so frightened and the only thing I could do was ask God by faith "Who am I, What is my purpose, Where did I come from and if I die I don't want to go to hell; I want to meet You (my Creator) face to face." From that point on that's how I learned more about me, my purpose and learn the Person that created me and now trying the preparation for going back to my Creator (by reading his Word, praying, Praising God and Worshiping Him; hoping to be accepted back to Him, when my journey is finished here. Nothing else makes sense anymore! Especially now that you are leaving. You made the time possible for me to read, pray, praise and worship by allowing me to retire. I will be forever beholding to this great Dr. Gardner.

People, places and things are temporary in the earth realm so I must hold on to eternity.

Looking at my scar reminds me every day how blessed I am to be alive and have had such good care. Even Dr. Jenkins that you recommended is still taking excellent care of me. I still have the port a cath a foreign object in my body for life time because it was so hard to put in that I would dare not take it out. I believe I almost died having it put in but there again God stepped in and again He stepped in when a nurse gave me an overdose of pain killer and my heart nearly pounded out of my chest after surgery. I have been through a lot and I won't complain but I'll always be thankful.

Let's face it, I depend on your opinion(s), your concern(s) for my wellbeing so much that I forgot this would be temporary yet I must say I am happy departing is in this life and not death. I have to try (with the help of God) to go on. I have a mammogram due December 14th and I will certainly have to have faith when someone new will read my results. I will get through it, but you sort of understand.

Do you remember after my surgery how frighten I was to touch my scared body or let you take the bandages off and I was so frightened of every intern and person except you? I trusted you because Dr. James recommended you and said so many great things of you character and Dr. James had my mother as a patient and he was and is a friend to my dear mother in North Carolina. You have proven to be all he said and some more. You took the staples out and I was so terrified yet you assured me it would not hurt and it didn't, the I was not lifting my arm and doing the prescribe exercise to get to the point to lift it and finally you yelled at me and said, "I have never messed up a patient's arm and you are not going to be the first." I promised I would do better and I did. You told me "take one day at a time" and I still do. Whenever I start stressing I think about you saying, "keep as much stress out of your life as possible" and I do. If it was not for you I would be forced to go back to work and just die because my family life is so stressed. Thank you again. Even again and again you did wonderful things for me as a patient. Remember, my husband and I were dislocated workers in the mist of this all, but you said, "if I didn't have health insurance just let you know and you would speak to some of my doctors to make sure I would have medical treatments". To God be the Glory for the good things that He has done through you. Those are just a tip of the iceberg concerning what you did as a faithful good practitioner and surgeon.

The word "tribulation" refers to all kinds of trials which may press in upon us. This includes such things as financial or physical need, trying *circumstances, mistreatment, or loneliness. In the mist o these afflictions God's Grace enabled and enables me to seek His face more diligently and produces in me a persevering spirit and character that overcome the trials and troubles of life. Instead of driving me to despair and hopelessness, tribulations brings forth perseverance, perseverance brings fort proven character, and proven character results in mature hope that I will not be disappointed. God"s Grace enabled me to look beyond my present problems and have hope and not weak faith to cause me to doubt, also allowing me to stagger not at the Promises of God through unbelief, but I am strong in faith, giving glory to God; and I am fully persuaded that what God has promised He is also able to perform. If I truly believe this Dr. Gardner then I can accept your retirement but it's still gonna be hard. I feel like I am losing a best friend in my life yet I have to accept the changes in life. Thank you and I wish special blessings in your life, something real special and you will know the blessings are unusual and from the Great Beyond. I really think you are too young to be retiring but who am I. (Smile) Your good deeds certainly speak for you. I am crying so hard now because I don't want you to go yet I know you should go and be with your family. Sylvia said I would be a basket case and she was right. But do you really know how much you* helped me in my life experience (of near death) to be a total being again after the most devastating, crises that one could face early in life? No you really don't! Don't even try to know. Just know all you have done is not in vain. Thanks.

Enjoy!

Mary E. Jones September 25th 2000 I will be a ten year survival cancer patient. Glory! Totally Amazing!

10 May 1999

Dear Dr. Gardner,

Words are not enough to express our deep gratitude to you! It was unfortunate that our mother discovered that she had breast cancer in a foreign land half a world away from her husband, at a time when she proposed in her heart to come and take care of her beloved grandson. However, where else could she find such a respectable and compassionate doctor like you? She stayed here for the surgery because she was touched by your kindness and trusted you when she met you, even though she didn't understand the language here. Not only is she haled physically and free of tumor, but she is also emotionally healthy because she has been very comforted by the continued act of your kindness to her, which she wouldn't ever dare to wish for even in her homeland.

Thanks so very much again for what you've done for us. Our father back in China also asked us to express his great appreciation to you.

If you ever have a chance to come to China, please stop by to visit our parents who live only 45 minutes from a very beautiful city called Hangzhou. We are sure they will be most happy to treat you to the best food and show you around.

Gratefully,

Ping Kaves Nu

www.ingramcontent.com/pod-product-compliance
Lightning Source LLC
Chambersburg PA
CBHW071300220526
45468CB00001B/216